Health matters

Exposing and correcting misguidance
Balancing and enhancing your health

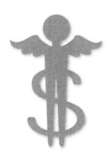

Neil Moffatt

First published in Great Britain 2011

Health Matters copyright © 2011 by Neil Moffatt

All narrative and diagrams © 2011 Neil Moffatt

ISBN

Table of contents

One	Who would mislead us?	1
Two	How they mislead us	7
Three	The simple truth	16
Four	The spanner in the works	25
Five	Prevention, cure and treatment	38
Six	Taking control of our health	45
Seven	Taking control of our food	54
Eight	Food advice for the masses	59
Nine	From the soil beneath our feet	71
Ten	Native diets	78
Eleven	Nutrition and digestion	74
Twelve	Low carbohydrate diets	98
Thirteen	The benefits of exercise	111
Fourteen	Injury and illness	118
Fifteen	Rest and relaxation	126
Sixteen	Meaning in life	137
Seventeen	Happiness	142
Eighteen	Force of habit	151
Nineteen	Attitude to self	160
Twenty	The wrong kind of thinking	171
Twenty One	Fear, anxiety and panic	179
Twenty Two	You cannot control the World	186
Twenty Three	Ego	199
Twenty Four	Compassion and kindness	210
Appendix One	My own health policies	216
Appendix Two	Précis of this book	225
	References	235
	Index	257

Credits

Serif PagePlus X4 software for making the design of this book a breeze

Steve Hemingway in England,
Esther Reiley, Beverley Winn, Kevin Arscott in Wales and
Tomáš Pavelka in the Czech Republic
for proof reading

Also by Neil Moffatt

Balancing Act
A short story with a moral twist

Learn Go
A beginners guide to the Oriental game of Go

Games of Go
A dozen fully commented games of Go

Go by example
Correcting mistakes in double digit kyu play

The purpose of this book

Your health is affected by a large range of factors, from physical welfare to aspects of the mind. Whilst there are many books that cover this multitude of health matters, there are few that try to provide a broad, balanced guide to your health. This book attempts to do just that.

It is therefore somewhat ambitious in its aim, and cannot of course hope to do any more than scratch at the surface of the health spectrum. The aim, therefore, has been to focus on those aspects of health that are likely to yield the most benefits for most readers.

However, before covering health benefits, I felt it vital to address the matter of health misguidance. For various reasons, especially influence and manipulation by industry, we are often not given the best advice for our health. Explaining why and how we are misguided and manipulated leads to a key tenet of the book – that our health is very much our own responsibility. By letting others determine our health, we allow it to be compromised.

Covering a range of physical, mental, emotional and spiritual topics, the book provides a broad awareness of the many factors that contribute to good health. The hope is that each reader will find a few aspects of their health that would benefit most from attention. The guidance offered should help create improvement in each chosen area, balancing out overall health, with the references providing routes to deeper understanding. At the very least, I hope that this book can be a catalyst to better health.

Note on references

I break with tradition and use a 2 character code instead of a number for book references. This is in part because references to the same book appear multiple times. But it is also because I believe a mnemonic is simply better than a number.

Chapter One

Who would mislead us?

It is patently clear that many of us struggle to achieve and sustain good health. We may over-indulge or simply fail to choose a healthy lifestyle. But in reality, even those who try to live healthy lives are often misinformed about what actually constitutes good health. I believe that there are two questions that have to be asked with regard this subversion of our health. Who would want to mislead us? And what do they have to gain by misleading us?

Because health covers a wide spectrum, good health is one in balance across that spectrum. By undermining some parts of the spectrum with misinformation and manipulation, the balance of our health is compromised. I expose these distorting influences as the opening gambit in this book for obvious reasons, but also for practical ones as well. This is because the advice I offer sometimes contradicts the conventional wisdom. Misinformation has manifested itself as wisdom.

Some of the ways in which we are mislead on health matters is in fact truly scandalous. Yet much that is potentially damaging to our health is offered in full knowledge of that potential. So I have to start by asking what kind of person would knowingly mislead us in a way that is deleterious to our health?

They would presumably not care about the effects of their actions. But how could such callous people actually get into a position with enough influence to adversely affect the health of many people?

You would assume that the kind of person intent on instilling harm on others would most likely be on the fringe of society, a part of the criminal fraternity. But manipulation of others is widespread, covering all walks of life, and certainly not limited to the criminal community. Yet most people try to put such miscreants out of their minds, truly believing that they *only* exist in poorer communities. They fail to recognise quite how many have actually risen to positions of influence. And that some can therefore mislead and manipulate millions of people with regard to their health.

Upbringing and circumstance can indeed draw certain types of people towards an anti-social lifestyle, and to develop a callous nature. For some, it is so much a part of family life that it is a natural route to take. However, genetics can have a more powerful influence on behaviour. It can predispose people to a socially dysfunctional life in a manner strong enough to resist all corrective efforts by their parents. (And sadly, these parents often then regrettably and mistakenly blame themselves for the anti-social behaviour of their offspring).

One such genetic profile is psychopathy, an anti-social mental illness that is characterised by a lack of conscience. Psychopaths are so short of, or even bereft of, the sense of conscience that socially unacceptable or destructive behaviour is an almost unavoidable consequence. Their genetic inheritance actually deprives them of the emotional tools required to care about the consequences of their actions. However, the majority of us only see the stylised and narrow movie representation of psychopaths as cold hearted and ruthless killers. Whilst some psychopaths are in this minority, the majority express their condition in less obvious ways.

Although the figure varies from book to book, it is generally believed that some level of psychopathic behaviour may be present in as many as 1 in 30 people. Affecting men more than women, in a football match with 30,000 spectators, for example, there are likely to be hundreds with psychopathic tendencies. Hardly a tiny minority, with the level of anti-social behaviour witnessed at some matches a testimony to that.

Psychopathy is more prevalent even than schizophrenia and bipolar disorder. Yet the image of the psychopath as a killer actually serves to blind us to the widespread prevalence of psychopaths in general society. We are also largely unaware of psychopaths in our midst because of the manner in which they disguise themselves, using charm as a smokescreen.

Whilst it is a mental disorder, the principle problem with psychopathy is that it has a devastating effect on family, friends, co-workers and society. Yet psychopaths regularly enjoy the fruits of their misbehaviours with minimal personal repercussions, and precious little guilt or remorse. They tend to be impervious to what little backlash does arise. It is a mental illness that it almost unique in that the 'suffering' is not incurred by the person with the 'illness', but by those around them.

This disorder was poorly documented until Hervey Cleckley published his authoritative treatise, "*The Mask of Sanity*" MS in 1941. In addition to profiling psychopathy, Hervey supplied highly detailed case studies that illustrated the diversity of the condition. So diverse in fact, that it became quite clear how difficult a condition it is to detect.

Essentially, psychopaths lack an array of emotions that normally temper behaviour in the 'normal' (neuro-typical) person. Psychopaths are principally devoid of conscience, worries and fears, and are thus frequently liberated to go out and grab whatever pleases them in the world. They are essentially uninhibited, unaffected by the feelings of regret, remorse and sympathy that bring the rest of us down to earth, keeping in check any potential anti-social behaviour.

Part of our failure to detect psychopaths is that the majority of people are socially adapted to give the benefit of the doubt to new people they meet. For psychopaths, we subconsciously fill in their emotional shortcomings. By the time we realise that we have encountered a 'bad egg', we have often been compromised by them, and they have moved on to their next victim.

Given enough time and exposure, however, psychopaths can be found out to be the rogues they are, and be treated accordingly. The smaller the community they are in, the more likely this is to be the case. When their audience is small, advantages taken of the trust that most people instinctively give to them is more clearly visibly. Their ability to charm their way back into favour is eventually eroded away.

One form of community is of course the workplace, varying in size from a one man start up to a sprawling international corporation. The bigger the company, the greater the scope for psychopaths to seek the anonymity that allows them to thrive undetected. The principle workplace attractions for the psychopathic mind are necessarily those that suit its peculiar traits. Not only do large companies offer the size that gives psychopaths the anonymity they need, but they also offer much greater potential for power, status and financial reward. Additionally, larger organisations tend to provide much greater novelty and variety, which suits their thrill-seeking nature.

With the acceleration of business competitiveness, change is a central issue, making speed, adaptability and risk-taking key survival factors. Psychopaths do not fear change and risk-taking, partly because they do not feel 'fear' in the general sense anyway. They relish both the novelty that accompanies change, and the opportunities that comes from the abandonment of some rules that is necessary to facilitate risk-taking. As they gain a reputation with management as a bold, fearless future star, they can be swiftly promoted through the ranks, often callously snubbing the colleagues they had recruited along the way to help them achieve their aims.

The path I describe can eventually take psychopaths to positions of great power and influence. They are very comfortable exercising this power, delegating to their minions, and doing whatever it takes to retain their new status. The success of the company is a key component of their success of course, so they are very happy to do whatever it takes to propel the business, and hence themselves forward. For example, to take the economical route of discharging waste products into rivers, rather than spend money on their safe treatment. To use sweatshops in Asia rather than provide a decent wage and working conditions. Even to engage in fraudulent accounting. In essence, they are happy to take the easy route of doing whatever it takes to maximise success at the expense of others. They literally transfer to the business their own reckless personality. Their anti-social tendencies are amplified and now operate on a much larger scale. Yet the absence of conscience blinds them to the impact of their actions, just as the thrill of success also blinkers them, (much as it often also does in non-psychopaths).

I guess you can see where I am going with this narrative. So far, I have generalised about the nature of these businesses and the roles that psychopaths play. It is highly likely that psychopath personality traits were in part to blame for the 2008 banking failures that brought about a global economic crisis. The problem had essentially been started by widespread, irresponsible selling of mortgages to those who could not afford to pay. It is likely that some of the bankers involved in this risky business were psychopaths. Certainly, when interviewed, many bankers saw no reason for guilt, or were un-moved by all the fuss, demonstrating a telling lack of conscience.

In the 'business' of politics, it is clear that some politicians exhibit psychopathic traits, not least in their blatant and repeated failure to directly answer questions put to them. Their focus of concern is for their own image and agenda, even though they are actually employed to serve others.

Ultimately, corporations have become the perfect vehicle for psychopaths to flourish. And it is important here to cover a little history to explain why. There were two connected problems with corporations that reared their heads in the mid 19th century. Firstly, when corporations failed, as they often did, the shareholders took the brunt of the costs, with many losing their homes and livelihoods as a consequence. Secondly, corporations were multiplying at such a rate that they were starting to look beyond business investors and towards the general public for investment. Shareholder limited liability was introduced to tackle both of these problems – corporation failure meant that shareholder loss was now limited to just the value of their shares, so the general public could now safely buy shares.

But as the average shareholding reduced, and the ownership spread geographically, the influence and control of individual shareholders on a corporation was reduced. To attempt to correct this, it was decreed in the late 19th century that a corporation was now to be treated as a person in their own right, independent of shareholders, management and workers. Corporations were to be independent entities, beholden solely to their shareholders and affiliated to no one person or persons. Joel Bakan recognised exactly what this meant in the subtitle of his book : "The Corporation : The pathological pursuit of profit and power". [CO] Corporations were adopting a pathological nature. One that was to prove unhealthy for the rest of us.

The corporation is in effect required, by law, to put the interest of its shareholders before anything else, including morals and ethics. In a sense, governments let the public down when they created the concept of corporations. What exactly were they thinking when they gave corporations the *mandate* to put money before people and the environment? Corporations are obliged, *by law*, to be *above the law*, if they can get away with it in order to give shareholders bigger dividends. They are not allowed to take an ethical stance if it compromises their profitability or shareholder status. Just ponder the consequences of this on the health of the planet and of the people living on it.

As these liberated corporations grew to monstrous sizes, they often ruthlessly used their power to feed this growth and simultaneously keep their shareholders happy. As mentioned before, corporations happily engage in anti-social practices when it serves them *practically* and *financially* to do so. If a large amount of money has been invested in a new drug, for example, the corporation producing it will probably seek to cover up any shortcomings in the performance of the drug in order to protect sales. Note also that if malpractice is in fact discovered, it is the *corporation* that tends to take the blame, and not the directors or managers. They merely operate it – the corporation is independent of them.

And this is the perfect environment for risk-taking, high-flying psychopaths to operate in. A corporation responsible only to shareholders, driven at least in part by psychopaths, is a potentially anti-health business. It is more likely to focus more on the business revenue from customers than on any consequential loss or damage to the health of those customers.

Chapter Two

How we are mislead

One emergent consequence of the growth and dominance of corporations is how they increasingly subvert and control the masses to suit their own obsessive and ravenous appetites for growth and profit. As the saying goes *"Power corrupts. Absolute power corrupts absolutely."* I'll set some of the groundwork of this mass subversion in this chapter, and cover some less obvious areas of influence in the next few chapters.

It should be noted that there are of course parallels between corporations and governments. In spite of any early honourable intentions, the acquisition of power often pushes some members of an elected political party to place the perpetuation of their power ahead of the need to serve the people who elected them in the first place. Both corporations and governments appear content to use their power to manipulate and subvert the masses. I discussed psychopathy to make it patently clear that certain human types are more than happy to exercise and wallow in such power for self-serving needs. The problem is that the sheer size and power of these corporations amplifies and extends the anti-social habits of the psychopaths employed within them. Corporations become a vehicle for psychopathic expression. In a broad sense here, man is his own most dangerous enemy. A small minority negatively impacts upon the many. But the biggest danger is not so much that they do this, but that they mostly do so using techniques that *hide* the damage they inflict. And much of this damage is to our health.

The first chapter of this book established *why* our best interests are not always at the heart of those who are in positions of control. Now I will discuss the techniques those in control use to mislead and manipulate us, along with our vulnerability to such influence.

In many ways, humans are like sheep. [IR] We are social creatures, heavily influenced by social conventions and by the inertia of thoughts and behaviours that get adopted as conventions by those around us. Social pressure steers our actions much more than we generally realise. We happily lie for social reasons, so can readily be lied to, or misguided, and rarely notice. Compounding this vulnerability is that we are not entirely in as much control of our faculties as we believe we are. [IR] The Economist magazine exposed the alarming way in which we delude ourselves in an article appropriately titled *"The conceit of deceit"* (27/Oct/2009 edition). It explained that if we act in a way that is obviously unacceptable, either to ourselves or to others, we will often unknowingly *fabricate* a reason that is acceptable, as a scapegoat for our real intent. Even when told that we are denying our own real intentions, we can be genuinely surprised, because we simply fail to recognise that a lot of our decision making is carried out by the subconscious.

Most of us take the normal path of accepting that things in life are as they are, have probably been as they are for a long time, and are therefore not to be questioned. We generally accept many things on face value, especially when these things appear to have always been that way. This leaves us vulnerable of course to manipulation. For example, it is widely accepted that because children love sweets that it is natural to give them sweets. It is such a prevalent habit, at least in the UK and US, that we are almost socially bound to perpetuate it. That children are often adversely affected by sweets, often making them hyperactive, is actually seen in a positive light – that they need the sweets to sustain these energy levels. We perpetuate myths in ways like this because it is the easy route to take, reinforced by the majority of those around us. We also invite the danger of marginalising our children if we deny them their sweet treats. And the children themselves likewise use social convention to insist that they do not miss out.

Yet research indicates that the situation is a catch 22 one – the very action of giving sweets to young children creates the taste for more. It is a vicious cycle. I do not know anyone who went without large quantities of confectionary when young, but I can readily testify to some of the damaging effects of refined sugars on my own health. Most obviously massive tooth decay, leaving me with a mouth full of mercury fillings, and the nasty prospect of mercury leaking into my bloodstream. But less obviously, osteoarthritis of both knee caps is highly likely to have been caused by the excessive sugar intake. And nutritional imbalances are also indicted in my hypoglycaemia (low blood sugar, as opposed to hyperglycaemia – high blood sugar – a more dangerous condition that diabetics regularly have to contend with).

Bad ideas can become established as the norm because they become reinforced by natural acceptability (sweets do of course taste nice), the breadth of uptake, and the passage of time. 'Established' norms are very hard to budge. When creating their own messages for the masses, governments and corporations supplement this combination of penetration (scale of audience) and duration (period of repetition) with *intensity*. They ensure that the message is strong and clear. Sadly, even if an idea is ill-founded, repeated promotion of the idea will eventually help gloss over its defects, critical though they appear to be to the validity of the idea. As the saying goes, *"Tell a lie often enough and it gets accepted"*. Governmental advice about our health is often misguided, but they repeat the messages so strongly, so often, and for so long, that the messages stick, and gain an unquestioned authority.

When delivering messages to the masses, those in power also swiftly recognise the importance of clarity and simplicity. They do so for two principle reasons. First, that to reach the masses, you must be able to reach across a wide spectrum of personalities and levels of intelligence. So a diluted, simplified message – a lowest common denominator – will maximise adoption. Second, that a simple message is most likely to be remembered, accepted and implemented. Simple messages carry an air of authority, especially when delivered powerfully. However, the world is a complex place, and simple solutions are more often idealistic than practical. This and other shortcomings in their method of influence will be covered in more detail in the next chapter.

Government and industry characteristically also use deflection to satisfy their agendas. They steer us in the wrong direction, hiding their true intent. Large corporations might promote a social conscience in full page adverts, yet spend a tiny fraction of money on good deeds. They paint a rosy picture as a smokescreen to distract us from the true reality of their operations. As already mentioned, politicians are famous for deflecting questions with questions. Or simply by just rambling on so long that the question is forgotten.

For example, here in the UK we have a serious and growing problem with young people drinking alcohol to excess. I wrote to the government asking why supermarkets are permitted to sell alcohol at below cost price. I expressed the view that this exacerbated the drinking problem. It made for easy access to cheap alcohol. And the sheer presence of so much alcohol on display sent the message to youngsters that alcohol has a similar status as foodstuffs – that it is perfectly normal to buy and consume large quantities. The question as to why the alcohol is available at below cost price was not answered. Instead, the reply from 10 Downing Street used deflection. If prices were raised, they claimed, the majority of moderate drinkers would suffer and be priced out of their healthy consumption levels. Deflection that detracted from the real problem, making the listener feel guilty for requesting a change. At the time of writing, alcohol is at its lowest price levels, in real terms, for decades. A price raise would not so much penalise the masses as see them paying fairer prices rather than the current perpetually discounted prices. So the deflection was a red herring.

By deflecting away from the reality of a situation, the government can avoid dealing with it, and the health of the British nation continues to suffer as a result. But notice that the supermarkets are the original guilty party here, with the colossal multi-national Tesco (branded as 'Fresh & Easy' in the US) as guilty as any. They too use deflection, claiming that they sell responsibly to adults when questioned, yet in reality use low price alcohol simply as an attraction to get increased customer numbers into their stores. They care about revenue and profit, not the social damage that the consumption of large quantities of alcohol inflicts. Imagine if a representative from Tesco were to respond to an enquiry about low priced alcohol with :

"Of course, it is a company strategy to leverage new customers in with low priced offerings. Alcohol is one of the most effective attractions, and we care more about our turnover, profit and growth than the consequences to the health of our customers of such a practice."

We, the masses, are also vulnerable to indoctrination, not least the relentless drive by industry for us to be consumers of products that we often do not need. The media creates a never ending need for more, playing on social comparisons to fuel these 'needs'. It leaves us in a continual state of discontentment. We delude ourselves into believing that each new gadget will make us happy, forgetting how quickly the novelty actually fades away. We buy the latest fashions in order to keep up with social trends, often unaware of how carefully these trends are controlled by industry.

The US and UK in particular are consumerist societies, partly because their governments focus on the economy, and consumption of goods is a vital economic factor. They project the message that a buoyant economy is good for the health and happiness of the nation. Again, this is a message that has been pushed so hard and for so long that we rarely pause to question it. In 1999, the UK Prime Minister Tony Blair actually did. He bravely admitted that there was a poor correlation between wealth and quality of life, and that running a country with its economy as prime focus was not working. Wealth has risen enormously in the UK since the end of World War 2, but health and happiness levels have not matched the rise, and have in fact declined a little. Just reflect on this concept – a focus on the economy largely means a focus on industry – but a focus on happiness means a direct focus on the welfare of the people. Most recently, there is a little hope for better things – in late 2010, David Cameron, the head of the conservative party, declared a plan to account for the happiness of the people in addition to the economy. Good news indeed.

One principle reason that the economy is traditionally used as the criteria for governmental success is that it is easily measured. It is quantifiable, and hence a ready guiding measure. Happiness is much more elusive. It is more a quality than a quantity, and very much more open to debate. Fundamentally, focusing on the economy keeps things simple. But, as mentioned earlier, simplicity is not often the best for us. For example, a focus on economics means a focus on the costs of public services – if money can be saved, then maybe tax payments can be reduced. Lower tax rates are a simple message which we can easily visualise, and which will therefore be more readily accepted. The lower tax rates are at the cost of lower quality public services. However, we often suffer a greater dip in the quality of life from this public service degradation than we gain with the slightly elevated spending powers of the tax reductions. In Denmark, for example, taxes are very high, but the focus is on maximising the quality of public services and of the general quality of life. It's probably no small coincidence that the Danes have often been voted the happiest nation on the planet (although the relatively small disparity in earnings between the rich and poor in Denmark is another key factor in the general levels of happiness there).

Before I leave the subject of consumerism for now, it is worth mentioning that we actually prefer less than more, yet get bombarded with greater and greater product choices. Research has shown that when choosing from a large variety of one product type, we tend to become overwhelmed, and indecisive. By buying one from a range of many, we are in essence rejecting all the others, and we struggle to decide which ones to reject. We are uncertain that we have made the best choice. Likewise with a proliferation of television channels, there is the nagging feeling that there could be something better on another channel. This overloading damages our sense of well being with a subtle degradation to our health. Subtle but insidious.

As corporations grow to enormous sizes, their appetite can become voracious. In order to survive market and economic fluctuations, they embrace a multitude of strategies that can give them an edge over the competition, and deeper and broader market penetration. Some of these strategies 'bend the rules' to smooth the way to sustain growth and profit. It is not so much that any one practice deployed is a problem – more that the combined effect of all practices is akin to a corporation bulldozing a route to success, with scant regard to the devastation left in their wake. Devastation that often directly and indirectly affects the health of the masses.

Governments are a prime target of corporations of course. Governments stand to lose large tax revenues if corporations threaten to uproot, so tend to handle them with kid gloves. Corporations use this softly, softly handling to carry out extensive lobbying, for matters such as increased deregulation and greater tax concessions. Research has shown that lobbying effectiveness is proportional to the amount of accompanying financial payments. Alas, many government members are suckers, it seems, for financial sweeteners, which can pave the way to other corporate benefits such as subsidies and even law changes.

These are of course not trivial matters. The 2008 banking collapses might well have been avoided if the regulations and regulatory bodies had more clout. But governments appear to be as obsessed with corporate growth at any cost as the corporations themselves. The lust for money appears to blind those in power to minor details such as the selling of mortgages to vast numbers of people so poor that they had precious little chance of maintaining payments.

Some of the lobbying is more insidious, as covered in great detail in "Food Politics".[FP] From her time as nutritional adviser to the US Food Guidance bodies, Marion Nestle describes in great detail how the food industry influences matters such as the foodstuffs represented in the US food guidance pyramid (the UK equivalent is the Eat Well plate). She was under intense pressure never to marginalise any food types. The publication of one particular variation of the food pyramid was actually halted because of industry protest. This industrial influence now extends to the hijacking of advisory bodies, of which more later.

The obsession with control, manipulation and hijacking soon caught up with newspapers. Long term news reporter Nick Davies describes how many decades of quality reporting, and the methods underlying such, were rapidly eroded with the arrival of the likes of Rupert Murdoch [FE]. Davies says that two long standing and vital activities of newspaper reporters which upheld the quality of their work were dropped for cost-saving purposes. First that they should go out and seek out news first hand. To be there when the Beatles landed back at Heathrow. To visit the scene of a bank heist. To go into the community and dig out stories. And so on. Time consuming, but crucial reporter work. Second, to check on the validity of reported news. Again, a time consuming activity, but a dangerous one to omit. These were swiftly reduced to a bare minimum simply to minimise costs and thereby maximise profits. Money was now king – truth was a lowly second. The result is that most reporters are mainly office bound, little more than technical secretaries, taking prepackaged news items from 'the wire', a set of news sources, the famous of which being Reuters.

The denial of the time needed to attend news worthy events, or to vet incoming news items left the door open for misinformation in its various guises to go to print. Big industry soon wised up to this, with burgeoning PR (public relations) departments creating press releases that placed their businesses in a favourable light. Much more dangerous, and very much more pertinent to a key theme of this book, is that the companies in the pharmaceutical industry started creating artificial ill-health stories, with remedies that involved drugs that they just happened to produce. The media has always been subverted for political purposes. Now it is being exploited by large corporations to suit their insatiable appetites for profit.

Industry is even not adverse to infiltrating sacrosanct domains such as education. The intrusion of soft drink vending machines in schools and colleges undermines the health of students in their formative years, often creating a lifelong habit for unwholesome drinks. The presence of the drinks in a school environment legitimises their consumption by association. At a deeper level, McDonalds has even managed to include a nutritional breakdown of a Big Mac™ in a school book covering food categories, purportedly to show 'all 4 food groups'.

More directly pertinent to health is medical care in the UK and US (and beyond), and how it has been corrupted and manipulated to suit both political and industrial agendas. This has been going on for decades now, so only the older amongst us will be fully conversant with the nature and scale of this erosion. Whilst it is patently true that the family physician in the early parts of the 19th century would have benefited from modern medical technology, practices and medicines, his approach was not swamped by these very same aids. These aids have taken the focus away from the patient as a person, making him more an anonymous vehicle for symptoms. They have also taken the focus away from some fundamental basics of health that I cover in the next chapter.

Chapter Three
The simple truth

It should be quite evident now that the truth about good health is often obscured by big industry. Alas, governments are caught up in this obscuration, partly under influence from industry, and partly because of the nature of politics itself, as you will shortly see. In summary, you are misinformed and mistreated by the big four : the pharmaceutical, food and medical industries and government (I refer to them as Big Pharma, Big Food, Big Medicine, and Big Brother). All have grown to be powerful, largely self serving institutions. We are tricked into seeing the *scale* of their authority as being proportional to their *degree* of value to us. They frequently create a common consensus of opinion that carries the weight of authority, but lacks an underlying concern for our welfare. [15]

It has to be admitted that the nature of politics does make the communication of meaningful messages to the masses difficult. Much as a school teacher aims to teach in a way that is well received across a range of abilities in a classroom, a politician advising on matters of health has to educate and inform across a range of intellects and backgrounds. But a whole nation is orders of magnitude harder to address than a classroom, so the messages necessarily get diluted down to a kind of lowest common denominator. They are diluted to be more simply understood, so as to be easily and universally applied. Coupled with this dilution is the need for message stability. It is crucial for leadership to present solid, simple and enduring messages for maximal acceptance and adoption.

One basic shortcoming of universal health guidance messages is that they necessarily fail to cater for the human diversity already discussed. Even diluting down to a low common level will fail to work for all of us. One size rarely fits all. Not only does the message lose strength by dilution, but for many, the message is in the wrong direction, simple thought the message may be.

An example will illustrate my point. For many years in the UK now, the Food Standards Agency (FSA) has advocated that we should all eat five portions of fruit and vegetables a day. A nice simple message. Except that it is overly simple. Is it really likely that five oranges a day is going to be as nutritionally sound as a mix of 3 different vegetables and 2 different fruit types? If your digestive tract is naturally a little too acidic, or too alkaline, the mix of fruit and vegetables you eat is either going to help or hinder your health. The necessary simplicity of the 5 portions message also fails to cover variations such as fruit and vegetable juices. Does a squeezed orange still count as one of your portions when liberated from the fibre that would otherwise make for a safer assimilation by the body? And what amount of spinach constitutes a portion? And quite where did the number five come from. Is it disastrous to fall short to four a day?

There is evidence to suggest that the number five was chosen arbitrarily – erring on the high side since most people would probably fail to achieve any target set as an ideal. Yet the message has been repeated ad infinitum, and has become a mantra for the masses as a consequence, to the point where it is actually socially unacceptable to question its validity. It is appalling to see young children drink a fruit juice in a cafe rather than eat whole fruit, or drink milk – a much better, but sadly less attractive alternative drink.

It should also be noted that vegetables are often bulky foods, and evidence points to the likelihood that such bulk can distend the stomach, with the consequent increase in the release of insulin by the pancreas in anticipation of large carbohydrate levels. [D1] Chronically high levels of insulin levels are not good for health, as will be covered in detail later.

More recently, UK and US governments have decided to accept the importance of omega 3 fatty acids, as commonly found in fish such as salmon, tuna and mackerel. This is essentially very good news, as they have wised up to the plethora of research that backs up this advice. However, the message is too simple again. The salient point is less about how much omega 3 fatty acids we consume, and more about the ratio between omega 3 and omega 6 fatty acids in our diet. It is not enough just to eat more omega 3 fatty acids but rather that we should eat less omega 6 fatty acids. Unfortunately, the processed food industry has a preference for promoting vegetable oils, and these are rich in omega 6 fatty acids, providing one cause for the imbalance in our omega 3/6 levels.

At a more subtle level, the types of omega 3 fatty acids is as important as their quantity. Fish sourced omega 3 fatty acids are high in Dososahexaenoic Acid (DHA) and Eicosapentaenoic Acid (EPA). DHA is good for the nerves and the brain, and EPA is good for your cardiovascular health. These are the principle reasons for consuming fish oils. Alas, in 2009, the US FDA approved Genetically Modified (GM) soybean as a source for omega 3 fatty acids. These are omega 3 oils high in Alpha-Linolenic Acid (ALA), which is weakly assimilated by the body. So the simple message hides a deeper reality. We appear to be steered to consume foods enriched with healthy fatty acids, yet are once again let down by the food industry focus on profit. It is much easier to harvest soybean than salmon, so we get second rate omega 3 fatty acids.

In effect, health messages become dogmas. The sheer repetition over many years ingrains them. We become indoctrinated, ground down. Even if we begin to question this guidance, we mostly have lives that are so hectic that little time, energy or inclination is left over for us to research the truth. If we do find the time, we may well struggle to find the truth underlying the messages. The Internet is a fabulous research tool, but a consensus of opinion has to be gained via much searching to be sure of the truth. Even then, there is lingering doubt cast by web sites with conflicting messages.

If we do unearth a finding that is contrary to the commonly held health opinion, we then find ourselves in a minority – our new enlightenment is not shared by our colleagues. Existing opinion weighs heavily against our minority view. We underestimate the power of social conventions and persuasions at our peril. Even if we have some belief in an opposing opinion, we can doubt ourselves as a result of social influence. Taking it further and contesting advisory body health messages that you believe to be misleading is an even greater challenge, and too daunting for most. So the authority behind misleadingly simple health messages remains mostly unchallenged.

Another example of the inertia of long held views is shown by scientists when confronted by a challenge to an existing theory. This is especially so in the case of specialists, whose whole career rests upon the validity of existing theories. Any new viewpoint will often initially be attacked and refuted, and the scientist proposing it ridiculed, since it undermines years or decades devoted to the existing paradigm. Given enough accumulating weight of counter evidence, however, scientists will eventually start to explore the new viewpoint. But it can take decades to reach the point of acceptance.

Science has evolved an unquestioned level of authority that in many ways matches that of the Medical profession. The 'Scientific method' is held in almost sacred esteem. It is de rigour in the West (in the East, however, it is complemented by a practical, holistic set of philosophies and outlooks). One of the dangers inherent in the level of authority that the scientific method has acquired is that it is arrogant enough in its own importance to marginalise alternative methods of seeking the truth. Any method, technique, food or drug that has not been subjected to scientific assessment is deemed too risky to accept. This danger is often unwarranted, but in the realm of personal health, with all its inherent complexity, the scientific method is even less justified in this arrogance. Understanding our own body and what makes it healthy is much more suited to an empirical approach than a scientific one. And the empirical approach is one of three contestants to this scientific dominance :

- Anecdotal evidence
- Traditional evidence
- Empirical evidence

I'll deal with each of these in turn before comparing them with the scientific method.

Anecdotal evidence is generally proffered by individuals. Individual experiences, but nonetheless necessarily very real for that individual. An inherent danger with anecdotes is the tendency for embellishment and a general inaccuracy of reporting. And that the anecdotal experience often cannot be repeated, such as when Norman Cousins cured his terminal illness. [AI] Anecdotal evidence can also be readily misconstrued, where a benefit can be attributed to the wrong cause. In general, anecdotal evidence is best used as a starting point for evaluation. But it should not be as summarily dismissed as it currently is. Fortunately, the concept of laughter as therapy that Normans struck upon is far from laughable. Dr Margaret Stuber led a US research team that demonstrated that children who were provided a laughter inducing environment coped with serious surgery more effectively and recovered more quickly. The scientific method may have subsequently shown the power of laughter on healing, but it required anecdote to bring this therapy to light in the first place.

The anecdotal, or individual, experience may not readily transfer to a treatment or method of more global value, but as said before, one size rarely fits all anyway. If the medical community want to dismiss anecdote, then I wonder if it is prudent to do so, since a patient essentially brings anecdotal evidence about themselves to their doctor at each visit anyway. Maybe the attempt by the doctor to normalise their condition is evidence of a mindset that is dismissive of anecdote. A mind closed to new ways of healing. Will a doctor really believe that a change in your diet might have caused your condition, or will he simply prescribe a drug for the symptoms of that dietary change?

Traditional practices and treatments accumulate over decades and centuries. They are tried and tested, honed and tuned according to their efficacy and appropriateness. They often embrace naturally available foods and medications, discovering and sustaining a long term relationship between plants and man.

To quote Ivan Illich, traditional cultures teach good health in terms of many diverse factors :

"... eating, drinking, working, breathing, loving, politicking, exercising, singing, dreaming, warring and suffering"

and not in terms of the relationship between symptoms and drugs. Traditional remedies are open to degradation of course, possibly even starting as a myth in the first place, or losing accuracy with the passage of time. But western life has sadly seen the erosion of much that was probably of high real human value in the past. Small fragments persist, such as the value of the stinging nettle plant. But it is easy to see how the multiple medicinal properties of such a plant could be lost in time, obscured by the irritation of its sting.

Finally, it should be recognised that the empirical method is in a sense a variation of the scientific method. Both involve experiment and observation, although empirical observation and iteration pairing is generally seen as a less formal version of the scientific experiments that form the basis of the scientific method. For example, nutritionists observe the effects of various diet formulations over many years on many different subjects. They may determine relationships between certain types of people and certain diets literally empirically. There is no formal testing of a specific diet formulation using precise scientific experiment methods, but the sheer weight of observations allows a finer and finer tuning of conclusions. In a sense, a stream of anecdotes are used to create hypotheses.

Returning to the scientific method, it is appropriate to point out some of its shortcomings also. First, it generally deals with measurable, *quantifiable* matters, and these do not always relate well to the *quality* of health. It is limited further by a need for repeatability. Again, this is not so easy with health matters – even selecting the same group of test subjects for a repeat run of a drug test will not mean that they are in the same condition they were in for the first test. A new set of test subjects may yield very different results. So the results of scientific health testing

21

can only ever yield statistically meaningful conclusions. The cost and discipline involved in scientific testing often also limits the size of test subject groups, which lowers the value of the statistical results. There are, in addition, scientific studies that rely on subjects taking notes or completing questionnaires. Such studies still fall under the umbrella of the scientific method, but are exposed to inaccuracies of reporting. It has been shown that we may say one thing to look good socially but actually do something else. Yet such flaws are glossed over because they fall under the influence of the authority of the scientific method. I would make a stab at guessing that a nutritional adviser with decades of experience would be able to provide more sound nutritional advice than any scientific research that involved the use of questionnaires.

Far more insidious is the very common and widespread failing of logic when determining the conclusion of scientific studies. Namely, that a correlation between two things does not necessarily mean a causal relationship. [DD] This is especially the case for studies that have multi-factorial influences. For example, the low incidence of heart disease in Mediterranean countries is often attributed to the use of olive oil. Yet this is one food in many that are relatively unique to these countries. Studies may conclude a happier disposition for those who exercise the most. But does such a study determine that the exercise led to the disposition, and not that the disposition led to the exercise? Certainly, depression results in lower levels of exercise. In summary, be wary of scientific findings that confuse cause and effect.

The scientific method dismisses anecdote for its small group size, and bias in reporting. As mentioned above, dismissing new discoveries is unwise. Drug companies use the lack of scientific testing to dismiss many traditional remedies and treatments. There is a certain arrogance here – do it their way or you do not count. Is it not anecdotal that potatoes are good for you? Has science tested the safety and effect on health of all the foods we eat? The rejection of empirical evidence is in a sense an attack on the basis of the scientific method itself. The argument is that the empirical method lacks rigour. Indeed it does, but the scientific method has been shown to be lacking rigour also.

In summary, all 4 routes to knowledge about the world have their place. Sadly, there is a prevailing mindset that ignores the potential for progress if the scientific protocol is not followed.

There are additional dangers with the use of the scientific method for testing drugs. First, that corruption is rife in scientific studies. As mentioned before, drug trials often yield the results desired rather than the true situation. This is not an inherent fault of the scientific method, but reduces the trust that can be placed in its use for validating the safety and effectiveness of drugs.

Second, that there is also an intrinsic danger in the statistical nature of the scientific method that is rarely brought to light. Consider the results of a drug trial, where 70% of the drug taking group received an improvement in their condition, 25% saw no change and 5% had an impairment in their condition. As long as the success percentage was sufficiently in excess of the placebo group success value, then the drug would be deemed effective. If the side effects were deemed minimal in relation to the benefit, the drug would be deemed safe. A mostly safe and effective drug generally gets approved.

But consider the reality here. One person in four is likely to receive *no* benefit from taking this particular drug. And one person in twenty is likely to *suffer* as a consequence of taking the drug. But if the drug is indeed approved, how do you determine if you are in the wrong category? Do you really want to take a drug that has an adverse effect on the very condition it is supposed to be correcting?

By way of example, consider the extremely well established drug morphine, used to dull pain. The effect is not so much to reduce the pain, but to make the experience of the pain much more manageable. I recently spoke to a district nurse on the matter. It appears that there are occasional patients who simply do not respond to morphine. In some, morphine has an antagonistic effect. Yet morphine is an approved and accepted reliever of pain. However, the scientific method certainly has not *proven* that it will relieve pain in *all* who take it. Merely that it is statistically *likely* to relieve pain. If it fails to help you, then the anecdote that you are not relieved by the use of morphine is more real and true for you than the scientific validity of morphine as a pain reliever. Empirically, the nurse knew that some simply did not benefit from taking morphine. The scientific method often actually does show the validity of the empirical and anecdotal, but it uses statistics to ignore them. The statistics should actually be used to acknowledge them.

Unlike the empirical method, which investigates the fringe effects of a treatment, the scientific method is deemed to have completed its (statistical) job when the testing has been completed. It is, in a sense, reckless and certainly closed minded to fail to explore why the drug being scientifically tested might have a negative effect. It may well be that certain constitutions or pre-existing conditions react with the drug. These are called contraindications. They often rear their head after a drug goes to market, when consumers feed back the deleterious consequences of taking the drug. Those that are in addition to the noted contraindications are then deemed side-effects, however, and treated as marginal matters. What gets labelled as side-effects are often the symptoms of the action of a drug that is not only ineffective for a particular person, but downright damaging for that person.

There is a elegant example of a medication that can often fail to achieve its aim. It is the most widely self-administered drug in the world, yet it can cause internal bleeding in small doses, being antagonistic to the collagen in connective tissues. In even slight overdoses, it can kill. It also blocks vitamin C uptake in blood platelets. Yet it has been approved for general use. It is, of course, Aspirin. If you really feel you should get the benefits of aspirin, far better to seek out the traditional version – Willow Bark. Big Science, in its mechanistic way, discovered the 'vital ingredient' in willow bark as aspirin, and proceeded to synthesise it. Just as with the loss of the fibre in a fruit drink, so it is with aspirin. The collection of chemicals in willow bark make the aspirin within it safe for the body to assimilate. But Willow Bark is slow to harvest and awkward to package, falling fowl of the mandate of drug companies to prune costs in order to sustain growth and profit.

Chapter Four

The spanner in the works

I have not quite finished exposing the shortcomings of drug trials. And what I have to say would actually be quite amusing if it were not so alarming. It concerns that nasty psychological spanner in the works for drug testing – the placebo effect. Literally meaning 'I will please', the placebo is the name given to a tangible health gain that can happen when a person believes that they are being treated by a proven method. For example, when a sugar pill is supplied instead of a real drug tablet, the patient might gain benefit because of the power in their belief that they had been actually given the drug. The placebo illustrates the power of the mind over the body. Or more accurately, that the body allows the mind to have more influence on its operations than we might at first think possible or plausible.

Henry Beecher is generally seen as the first to bring the placebo concept to mainstream awareness. [PL] He was an American anaesthetist treating injured soldiers in the Second World War. On one particular day, he was presented with a patient who had especially serious injuries, and was necessarily in a great deal of pain. It was standard practice to reduce the pain using a morphine drip. Except that stocks of morphine had been depleted. Rather than disappoint the soldier, he decided to simulate the morphine administration, using a saline solution instead, hoping, with an insightful instinct, that at least meeting the expectations of the patient would be a calming influence. But he was surprised to find that the effect of the saline solution was much the same as if morphine had been given.

The power of expectation made an inert salt solution almost as effective at killing pain as a powerful drug.

The reporting of this story had a major impact on medical and other professions, as they swiftly sought to explore the ramifications. And the status of the placebo effect moved from dismissible anecdote to one of tangible importance. One of the most significant consequences of this newly found legitimacy was the eventual inclusion of a placebo group in scientific testing involving humans. And that included drug testing of course. Drug companies had a new adversary to contend with. The placebo effect proved to be a powerful opponent, even if it was still only treated as a fringe irritation that had to be accounted for.

Traditionally, top quality drug-testing was carried out using two groups – one taking the drug and one not taking it (although much testing still had no control group for comparison at all). With the introduction of a third test group, taking a placebo pill, it soon became clear that the sheer *expectation* engendered by the administration of drugs had been inflating the *value* of those drugs. The new test group meant that drugs had to stand head and shoulders above any placebo effect that was simply the result of being given some kind of treatment, bogus or not.

There was initial ethical concern that an additional group of ailing subjects were going to miss out on the value of the drug being tested. But this concern was swiftly alleviated when the majority of trials showed quite how consistently powerful the placebo effect was. The sheer matter of being attended to, even with a dummy treatment, was triggering the power of the mind.

The simple act of visiting your doctor can also kick start the healing process. More so if your doctor treats you in a positive, supportive manner. Even if he administers a placebo, your condition is highly likely to benefit. But not many doctors, it would seem, are happy to give out sugar pills. The ethics of doing so are questionable of course. So more often than not, the doctor will administer a drug, knowing that the administering of *anything* is crucial to the placebo role in the healing process. In a sense, doctors are trapped into taking some action, and we the patients seem to expect that action to be tangible, such as the material form of a drug. We want to feel to be doing *something* – to be active in resolving our condition.

In spite of this growing awareness, the placebo is still a much undervalued mechanism. Because it is often seen as an awkward interfering factor in drug testing, the scale of its power, and hence potential aid to good health is generally overlooked. That this happens is of course in part a result of its slippery nature – tell someone that you are giving them a sugar pill and the placebo effect is heavily reduced (but curiously enough, often not entirely lost). It is worth illustrating, however, the power of the placebo effect with some examples.

In 1950, the Journal of Clinical Investigation reported on a placebo trial carried out on 33 pregnant women, chosen because of their suffering with 'morning sickness'. [PL] They were administered a drug that they were told would stop their sickness. In addition to observing the effect of the drug, and listening to the feedback from the women, they also lowered an instrument down their throats that enabled their stomach contractions to be visualised. Sickness levels were almost universally lowered.

So how was this a demonstration of the placebo effect? It was in reality a profound demonstration, since the administered drug was not even a sugar pill. They were given a syrup made from the ipecacuanha plant root, normallly known to irritate the stomach lining and induce vomiting. Commonly known as syrup of ipecac, the women had been given an emetic, yet had experienced an opposite effect. The expectation given to the women by the researchers had reversed the effect of a powerful treatment. This is a profound finding, made many decades ago, yet seemingly put to one side as a mere curiosity. It is far too significant to be forgotten. It has recently been repeated with caffeine and caffeine-free drinks, and alcohol and alcohol-free drinks to the same counter-intuitive effect. Yet it is still not properly accepted, explored and exploited for more profound health benefits.

On a sadder note, the placebo effect has an opposite. The so-called nocebo effect. It is not hard to visualise the placebo effect as a subconscious fulfilling of wishful thinking – that the tablet you are being given will heal you, even if, unbeknown to you it is merely a sugar pill. By the same token, if we engage in negative expectation, the subconscious can fulfil this likewise. If you believe that you are too tired to do something, you are likely to become too tired to do that thing. Self-fulfilling prophecies as it were, in both cases, but in opposite directions. The placebo is a form of positive thinking or visualisation or expectation. The nocebo is negative thinking – embracing failure or disaster. These matters are covered in more detail later on in the book.

A very sad example that illustrates both placebo and nocebo is the case of a cancer patient of Bruno Klopfer, an American psychologist in the 1950s. He prescribed Krebiozen, a new cancer drug, to a patient. It worked very well, and the patient's tumours went into remission. But when the patient later read newspaper articles debunking the value of the drug, his tumours came back. Alarmed at this reversal, the wise doctor gave the patient a placebo. He described it as an enhanced version of Krebiozen. Of course, it was not exactly ethical to lie to the patient, but it was not exactly prudent to take punitive action against the doctor since the patient's tumours went into remission again. Sadly, the newspaper ran a subsequent article again dismissing the effectiveness of this drug, the poor patient bought into the negativity once again, and his returning tumours soon killed him. [PL]

On a lighter note, a more recent placebo test was carried out on the efficacy of ultrasound treatment on the reduction of pain following tooth removal. They discovered that the key factor was the application of the cream that the ultrasound device sat upon, rather than the device itself. After applying the cream, and then pressing the ultrasound device against it, the pain was relieved, *regardless* of whether the machine was switched on or not. Again, the expectation of pain relief brought about by the ritual was significantly greater than was actually delivered by the device itself. And there was a curious twist to this discovery. If they turned the ultrasound up towards its maximum power level, the pain relief was actually reduced.

There is another twist to the placebo effect that impacts on drug testing. It concerns the existing 'gold standard' drug trial, as characterised by the following main attributes :

- One set of patients receives no treatment.

- A second set of patients receives the drug being tested

- A third set of patients receives a sugar pill (placebo) that looks like the drug

- The trial is double blind – neither the patients nor the administers of pills know who is receiving the drug or the placebo

- The trial is randomised – the patients are randomly assigned into these groups

Key to the double blind aspect is that patients should not be able to differentiate between the placebo and the drug. Recent research with anti-depressant drugs showed that this is not the case. [PL, EN] It appears that many patients are able to work out which if they were receiving the drug, because they could detect the *side-effects* of the drug. They could sense that they were taking an active substance as opposed to a placebo pill. Research was carried out to try to cancel this detection process by using a drug instead of an inert placebo tablet. The drug would be one that generates similar side effects to the drug under test, but not any anti-depressant effect. The net effect was that the drug was no longer demonstrably more effective than placebo. Minimising the flaw of drug detection (that had negated the vital double blind aspect of drug testing), showed the drug to be much less effective as an anti-depressant.

To explain this, it appears that by being able to detect that a drug rather than placebo was being administered, the patient's expectations of healing would be elevated. Conversely, a patient that knew he was taking a placebo would have a reduced expectation, and hence lowered placebo effect. There is a profound conclusion to be drawn from this – that drugs shown in scientific studies to outperform placebo may actually have been operating *by virtue* of the placebo effect in *addition*, or *in place* of any biochemical effect. The existing gold standard drug trial is not as sound as it is made out to be.

And I have one more twist to offer. This one is by courtesy of the British 'New Scientist' magazine (Issue 2670, 20 August 2008). Researchers discovered that the effect of the anxiety reducing drug Diazepam virtually vanished when it was administered *unknowingly*. Likewise, it was discovered that morphine could be provided at fairly high levels to patients in pain with no effect on that pain if administered without the patient's knowledge. This too is a telling discovery. Morphine is an extremely well established and effective treatment for pain, effective in most people. Yet, it seems, a part of this very efficacy is due to the placebo effect. This links in well with the placebo detection problem – anti-depressant drugs being barely any more effective than placebo when the placebo used was indistinguishable from the drug.

But it is much more profound than this suggests, as Professor Irving Kirsch inadvertently discovered when he embarked on an exploration of the placebo effect. This was lucidly and succinctly detailed in his aptly titled book "The Emperor's New Drugs". [EN] Via meta-analyses of anti-depressant drug trials, he discovered that the drugs under test uniformly performed 25% better than placebo. This implied that the the advantage was caused by the chemical effect of the drug on the taker.

But when he dug deeper, he found that this 25% anti-depressant edge was in fact a super-placebo effect. When an anti-depressant drug is taken, via trial or in daily life, the side effects are the signal to the taker that the drug is doing something. The *stronger* the side effects, the stronger the anti-depressant effect on the taker. Just as larger placebo pills have a larger effect, so it is with anti-depressant drugs. We have evolved a belief that the stronger the medicine, the more effective it will be. When an analysis of Prozac, the most famous of anti-depressant drugs was performed, the correlation between the degree of side effects and the efficacy of anti-depressant action was almost perfect (it had a 0.96 correlation value). [EN]

It appears that there may be **minimal** or **no** anti-depressant effect attributable to chemical action by anti-depressant drugs. And this is a staggering conclusion. Step right back, and picture the reality of the situation. A drug such as Prozac, taken by millions, earning countless billions for the manufacturer, may simply be a placebo tablet. The effect felt is mostly a placebo one, that is actually enhanced by its side effects – the placebo effect is enhanced or caused by the damaging, unhealthy side effect actions on the body. This is a paradoxical, but deeply sad conclusion, and illustrates the degree to which our health can be and often is subverted by Big Pharma. A subversion assisted by the regulatory bodies, who even help to cover up the existence of negative drug studies.[EN]

As an aside, but important to note, it is vital to know that this does not imply that all drug trials are subject to such profound super-placebo effects. It appears that the placebo effect is most pronounced with pain and depression suppression.

The net effect of these findings is that the gold standard drug trial is seriously flawed. And the net effect of that is that there are likely to be drugs on the market that passed drug testing that would have failed such testing if the testing flaws were limited or removed. A proposed 'platinum standard' drug testing regime would supplement the gold standard as follows :

- The placebo should resemble the drug in side effects as well as visually. Or, alternatively, for the test subjects to *not know* that they are being involved in a drug trial. They would not then consciously or subconsciously scrutinise the tablet they are being given to see which group they had been assigned to.

- Have a fourth test group, where the subjects are administered the drug unknowingly.

Of course, the disguising of a placebo to resemble a drug in its entirety is a thankless and highly impractical task. And there are the ongoing ethical issues with the administering of sugar pills to patients who are told they are being given drugs. There may also be logistical difficulties hiding the administration of the drug in the fourth test group.

But the increased elimination of the placebo effect would most likely better vet the drugs being tested.

As things stand today, it appears that some of the drugs we are prescribed largely *rely* on the placebo effect for their own effectiveness. This is fine in one sense – we do want to get better after all. But if that could be achieved with a much cheaper placebo, or with the kind of mindset that is the underlying mechanism of the placebo effect in the first place, then much money could be saved. The likely consequence, it would seem, is that just as the novelty of taking the drug fades over time, the power of placebo fades likewise. As drug taking becomes mechanical, we forget precisely why we are taking a drug, and we fail to tell the body to act upon it. Coupled with the body's reduced response to drugs through habituation, it is no wonder that drugs lose their potency over time.

An investigation into the extent to which approved drugs relied on the placebo effect for their own effectiveness was reported in the February 2008 edition of PloS medicine. [HM] A meta-analysis of 35 trials of four major anti-depressant drugs, commonly known as Seroxat, Prozac, Effexor and Serzone revealed over 80% of their effect was attributable to placebo. This illustrates the degree to which drug trials can mislead.

Note also that drug companies also respond to the invasive nature of the placebo effect by running pre-trials. They use these to weed out the participants who show the strongest placebo effect. [HM] Whilst this might sound innocuous, it is hardly fair or scientific – the subjects thus recruited for the main trial have already been selected to favour the drug ahead of the 'inconvenient' placebo effect.

I have been curious about the placebo effect for many years now. But in all the articles on it that I had read until recently, there had been no discussion of any corollary of the placebo effect. Namely, why does the body wait for the brain to engage in the belief that enables and empowers the placebo effect? Why does the body not automatically heal in the first place?

To my mind, this is a deeply fundamental aspect of the placebo affect, and the lack of material on the matter is puzzling. However, I did eventually chance upon a brilliant essay on the placebo effect by the Scientist Nicholas Humphrey that explored this issue. [MM] I strongly urge you to read this essay, also obtainable for free as a pdf file on the Internet (It is entitled – "Great Expectations : The evolutionary psychology of faith healing and the placebo effect"). Whilst it fails to explain all facets of the placebo effect, it does have a strong ring of plausibility.

He uses exquisite logic to seek an explanation for the placebo effect by way of human evolution. He argues that it must have evolved to its current universal form for sound survival and/or reproduction reasons. In essence, he splits ailments that respond to the placebo into two categories. The first is the set of ailments that result from defensive action by the body. Randolf Nesse and George Williams say :

*"... those conditions from which people seek relief are not in fact defects in themselves but rather self-generated **defences** against another more real defect or threat".*

For example, pain is a response to injury, fever a response to infection, and depression a response to loss. Humphrey points out that these are *appropriate* and generally *beneficial* responses. In modern times, we do however seek to suppress or remove these beneficial symptoms, but are often unwise to do so. The second category is the class of actual injuries and organic sicknesses that we occasionally have to endure. Here, we refer to the role of the placebo effect in accelerating the healing process, rather than in suppressing the symptoms.

When we use the placebo effect on the first category, we expose ourself to complications. By reducing the pain that the brain creates in response to an injury, we risk an aggravation of the injury. If placebo lowers fever symptoms, we can feel well enough to get up and about, and slow the healing process by doing so.

For the organic ailments in the second category, placebo will appear to be a win-win situation, as healing is sped up, and we get back to full health faster. But it too has a side effect. The immune system is very expensive to operate at full power, especially if the diet is not furnishing enough of the right nutrients. Targeting the full weight of the immune system towards one particular ailment means that other parts of the body are being deprived of both immune system support and of general resources.

The underlying point here is that the body is involved in resource management. Historically, the body has build up a set of standard mechanisms for balancing resources, for example, keeping spare immune system on hold in case of future attacks that may be more important than the current problem. It acts in ways that have served humans effectively in a statistical sense over the centuries.

But there are times when it would make a better job of resource management if it knew when times were safe enough for the immune activity to be ramped up, and when times were hard so that it could start to divert resources to defence from predators and the like. There is evidence, however, that such indicators already exist. Immune system activity drops when we are stressed – stress being a good general guide to an environment requiring a defensive posture. And the immune system is bolstered by sleep and laughing – both signs that it is safe to lower the defences.

It appears that the planning and forecasting roles possible with the advent of higher brain functions in the frontal lobes are the key to the placebo effect. If we can forecast that all will be fine in the near future – if we believe that times ahead are likely to be safe – then the immune system can ramp up the healing process. But the body needs the brain to tell it of the forecast – it is like an army taking advice from central headquarters. Certainly, there are well documented pathways from the brain to the immune system that facilitate this communication.

Note, as a slight aside, that the body and its immune system shows signs of their ancient heritage when we get injured during sport. The pain we feel is heavily suppressed, because statistically speaking, those who were able to suppress pain when hunting for food were those more likely to make the kill and survive. The immune system has not yet caught up with modern times in this and other matters.

Returning to the subject of drug trials, I would say in summary that I recommend a cautious wariness of the efficacy of drugs. Rarely do drugs affect the one part of the body they are intended for, which in part explains the proliferation of side effects. But mainly because it would seem that many drugs are simply not very effective. The power of the mind – how you think – is a much more powerful deciding factor in your health. This will be a major theme of the latter part of this book – a kind of 'piece de la resistance'. For now, I can offer a taster of more to come in the form of self-fulfilling prophecies, a variant on both the placebo and nocebo effects.

I no longer recall the source of the information, alas, but post mortems on many sufferers of terminal cancer apparently revealed that the cancer itself was often not the main cause of death. There is one story that corroborates this, of a man diagnosed with terminal cancer, fading away into an ever weaker state in hospital. [SD] Very late in his decline, his wife received a nervous phone call from the doctor, apologising deeply about a huge mistake. They had informed the *wrong* man about the cancer. Within weeks of hearing the news, the man rapidly recovered to full health. He had been fulfilling the prophecy of the diagnosis, and then subsequently fulfilled the prophecy of a clean bill of health.

Self-fulfilling prophecies can be a form of placebo that can be a spanner-in-the-works for ourselves, rather than for drug companies. Their scope is not limited to the extreme situation I described above. They can and do pervade everyday life. To a very large extent, what we think defines what we are and what we will become. I remember after turning 30, that my speed around a tennis court started to decline. I obviously had it in my head that this was a pivotal age for decline in sporting capability. When I noticed, however, how closely linked the decline was to that arbitrary age, I realised that I was giving in to a general, but gradual loss of natural pace. So I decided to speed up. True, I had to push myself more than I had before to achieve this, but I have maintained an attitude of outperforming age related sporting expectations ever since. At the time of writing, I am 53 and still play soccer, preferring to play on the wing, where sprinting is a key part.

Although I have just related an anecdote, I hope that you can see its value. I will cite a controlled experiment on the matter as a counterpoint. It was reported by the BBC Horizon programme "Don't grow old : Genes vs Lifestyle" (first broadcast 9th February 2010). They described an experiment carried out in the 1970's with a group of men aged 75, each sufficiently immobile that they were normally attended to by a carer. Most were barely able to shuffle around. They were temporarily transplanted to a country house which had been decorated in 1950's style. Even the TV programmes were from that era. The idea was to attempt to both psychologically and physically transport these elderly men back twenty years. The physical side of the equation was that they would have to look after themselves. They were told to take as long as was needed, but that they would have to be self sufficient for the duration of the experiment, walking unaided, even up the stairs, cooking for themselves and doing all the cleaning.

Health measurements were made before and after the experiment. The net effect of the enforced increase of exercise and self sufficiency was not just a tangible increase in mobility. Their blood pressure was lowered. Their eyesight improved. And even their intelligence improved. These latter factors are generally recognised to be in irreversible decline at age 75. And how long did such an experiment have to run to achieve such benefits? Just one week.

Note that the separation of the elderly from their family is deemed to be the biggest cause of their illnesses, yet this is rarely recognised. Like the self-fulfilling prophecy that you will slow down as you age, this social aspect of ill health is too vague to be treated by drugs so mostly gets ignored. [LM] The unquantifiable does not fit well into the domain of scientific enquiry or scientific credibility.

A similar experiment was carried out by Harvard Scientists in 1989. They placed subjects aged 70+ in a retreat furnished to make their lives there look and feel like 1959. Ten days was enough in this retreat to improve the health of all, with some acting 25 years younger than their real age.

This paints two pictures – first that we allow ourselves to follow the normal course of events that society expects of us. And second, how a much better alternative path is available for remarkably little cost. We create our destiny, and an underlying message from this book is that the benefit to cost ratio of taking a better route for our health is high. I hope that I can not only make you want to take greater control of your health, but to stick at doing so.

At an even more every day level, if we anticipate difficulties, for example with a meal we are attending with friends, then difficulties are more likely to ensue, because our mindset is one that will enable what we expect. The reality is the one that we make. And this is the big point here – not only can we get misguided from the path to good health by big industry, but we can misguide ourselves. Misguidance in the subtitle of this book was intentionally ambiguous, and shows how it is a twin-edged sword.

To illustrate the degree with which we are vulnerable to suggestion, and hence misguidance, consider the outcome of the outstretched arm experiment. [FF] Subjects were asked to hold an arm outstretched in front of them, and told to repeat the words '*I am strong*' a number of times. The experimenter would then attempt, unsuccessfully, to push the outstretched arm down. When the exact same procedure was repeated, but with the words '*I am weak*', the result was very different. This time, the subject could not stop his arm from being pressed down.

This itself is an amusing outcome, but one made profoundly more so when the cycle of procedures was repeated again. Now, the subjects were aware of the link between the words and their resulting strength. But no matter what they did, their arm was always relatively weaker when citing the words '*I am weak*'. It therefore did not matter whether they believed what they spoke – the meaning of the words still filtered through to their subconscious. The concept of self-fulfilling prophecies is rather deep and pervasive, as you can now see.

Chapter Five

Prevention, cure and treatment

Physicians from earlier, 'primitive' times, worked more with a qualitative, holistic approach to health than they do today, acquiring decades of familiarity with each and every member of the families they served. They would know the typical response to stress and ailments of each of their patients, allowing any symptoms to be seen in the light of their constitution and their personal history. Because the physician was aware of the diversity of 'normal health' signatures, such as heart-rate, blood-pressure, body-weight and resistance to disease, he was able to take a more intelligent course of action, unique to each person. Modern practice has neither the time, nor the inclination to piece together a long-term picture of each patient, preferring instead to normalise treatment according to standard measures. In effect, to run medical treatment mechanically, out of tune with individual variance.

If my doctor measures my heart-rate and finds it to be 49 b.p.m., what is he to think? This is below 'normal', but only in a statistical sense – it happens to be perfectly normal for me. Conversely, a heart-rate of 75 b.p.m. at rest would be a little worrisome for myself, but would not solicit such concern from my doctor. This focus away from the person to a mechanised treatment of his symptoms is dangerous to the health of that person. This distancing from the patient is exacerbated by the modern un-empathic and un-sympathetic approach of modern physicians. The physician is king, 'owning' the treatment, often withholding the full story, especially the possible side-effect of administered drugs. Research has shown that patients treated with respect and who are well informed about their condition heal faster and need less medication. [SD]

On a deeper level, the passage of time has seen another diversion of focus. Fundamentally, good health should have *prevention* of ill-health as the prime focus. When this fails, attempts at *curing* the ill-health that arises should be made. It is only when seeking a cure proves elusive or protracted should the final course of action be made. Namely, to *treat* the symptoms of the ill-health. Today, medicine tends to work almost exclusively with this 'last resort' treatment phase. In addition, the focus on symptoms as the be-all and end-all of our health introduces two more problems.

First, that there is a tendency to see symptoms as entirely undesirable and unhelpful, and therefore to suppress them. This fails to address the cause, merely camouflaging the body's signals of distress. The condition continues unabated, and the lack of symptoms gives us both false hope and stops us dealing with the cause. If the cause is psychological, it may then seek an alternative means of expression via new symptoms. These are likely to get suppressed in turn, and a vicious, rather than virtuous cycle is engaged in, where a stream of symptoms are chased, and the underlying cause is left to fester and grow.

Second, that treatment by drug, rather than 'natural' remedy, can introduce imbalances in the body that can also manifest as other symptoms. These too can get chased in a similar vicious regression.

Knowing as you now do how callous big pharma can be in their pursuit of profit and growth, this repeat business of symptomatic treatment is fair game to them. It is significantly more important that revenue streams are sustained or expanded by dishing out more and more drugs than it is to cure the conditions themselves. To quote Anson Chi[YE]:

"No one talks of cures these days. Is it because a cured person is no longer a 'customer'?"

For the medical industry to focus on curing patients would be akin to shooting themselves in the foot. But worse still for these precious revenue streams would be to prevent these conditions ever arising among the population in the first place. By way of example, is it not better to build a house with a proper damp proof course than incur the disruption, aggravation and cost of remedying subsequent rising damp? But for a builder, this damp iwould be seen as welcome extra work and income. The problem we have today is that we are much more likely to treat symptoms in such a way, rather than their cause. Is it not wiser to retrofit a damp proof course rather than dry out the affected walls and paint over with damp resistant paint? Alas, even respected businesses focus on treatment rather than prevention or cure. The multi-billion dollar cancer industry spends a pittance on cancer *prevention*. By preventing cancer in the first place, it would largely put itself out of a job. (Not only that, but it should be pointed out that some cancer drugs are actually carcinogenic in addition to their well known immunosuppressive effect [SD]).

The point here is that prevention is by far the most intelligent, practical and cost effective way to handle human health, with cure a poor second, and treatment a weak third. It is truly criminal how prevention has universally acquired a weak reputation, and how it has also even been suppressed.

We live in a society that is more reactive than pre-emptive. When a fireman rescues people from a flaming office block, he is lauded as a hero, but the person who ensures that the fire extinguishers are operational is never given such accolades. In his efforts to prevent a fire, he is actually treated negatively as a fussy busy-body, and often denied the time to carry out his checks. Preventing a fire is rarely treated with the same scale of importance as rescuing those subsequently trapped in a flaming building without functional extinguishers. This hopefully illustrates the blind-spot that humans seem to have with the reality of preventative measures.

One of the reasons that prevention is not well embraced is that the end product of preventative action is often a non-event. You prevent a negative outcome that may or may not have happened anyway – fire extinguishers may be checked regularly for decades and never be brought into service with a real fire. Because we often cannot relate back the *lack* of tangible consequences to the *action* we took, we question the *value* of that action. Prevention often acquires its poor reputation by virtue of this weak feedback – humans operate much better with a simple cause-effect pairing.

But there are preventative actions that we *can* adopt whose effect can be more easily felt. For example, where there is an ongoing or repetitive compromised health factor, such as that which comes from chronically poor sleeping patterns, we can take action to prevent future incidences. If we stop burning the candles at both ends of the day, for example, we prevent poor sleep. This creates a virtuous cycle of behaviour because cause-effect feedback is present. It may have a poor reputation, but prevention is a very important, but much neglected subject, a situation I hope to remedy a little in this book.

When ill-health is established rather than prevented, the modern focus on symptoms is at least partly correct. But we are all different, with different lifestyles and medical histories, and the modern obsession with symptoms often fails to take these into account. The symptoms of ill-health are rarely sufficient on their own to allow an accurate diagnosis of the *cause* of that ill-health. A pain in a knee, for example, may be a referred pain – one that results from a problem elsewhere in the body. A trapped nerve, or hip weakness may be the original cause. In such cases, treatment may be required both for the cause *and* the referred knee damage. However, the medical profession is financially constrained, and also subject to intense pharmaceutical influence, so rarely has the time or mindset to make a proper diagnosis. For the purposes of economy and efficiency, there is a growing tendency to see a one size fits all treatment methodology. For each symptom, one drug is deemed appropriate, with alternative drugs simply variations of that theme. The shortfall in diagnosis is therefore multiple :

- Too little is known about the history and lifestyle of the patient
- Too little time is spent searching for the source of symptoms
- Symptoms are treated as universally consistent in etiology, with a uniform treatment mistakenly assumed appropriate

41

G. T. Wrench M.D. provided a powerfully persuasive argument against symptom-only medicine in his description of the effect of one nutritional shortcoming in laboratory rats. [WH] He described research that involved no less than 2,243 rats along with some other animals. They were provided with a diet acutely short in Vitamin A, necessarily resulting in many illnesses. It is the sheer number and diversity of these illnesses that is the moot point of their findings. These ranged from bronchitis, pneumonia and diarrhoea to nasty matters such as inflammation and the degeneration of nervous tissues. If you or I were to present any one of these conditions to a modern physician, they would rarely diagnose the cause correctly. (This is especially true with nutritional shortcomings in fact, since Medical school tends to treat nutrition as a minor factor in human health). Most dangerous is the common practice of assigning one drug per symptom, which can be seen as obviously flawed in the light of this research. Not only will treatment of the *symptoms* have little chance of remedying the *condition*, but the condition could be *exacerbated* by drugs used in this treatment. And this is not a matter of side effects – here I am talking about the principle effect of the drug working in the wrong direction for an ailment because of a failure to diagnose the true cause of the ailment.

Part of the difficulty in the diagnosis of ill health is the degree to which human biochemistry differs. Not only can symptoms express very differently because of this diversity, but treatment should, but rarely does, take into account how very different we are from each other. As Hippocrates said :

"*... more important to know what sort of patient has a disease, than to know what sort of disease a patient has.*"

Roger Williams, a 27 year old man, was administered morphine as a sedative after undergoing an ulcer operation. But it had an opposite effect, not only depriving him of sleep, but significantly unsettling his mind. So the Doctor increased the dose. The result was disastrous,

Williams saying that "...[I] *nearly lost my mind"*. The unexpected nature of his reaction to morphine drove him to embark on research into human diversity, as recorded in his 1956 book "Biochemical Individuality". [BI] He discovered many curiosities that collectively make us possibly more internally variant than externally.

By way of example, the base of the stomach can apparently be sited between 1 and 9 inches below the base of the sternum. Resting heart-rates in normal, healthy men can range from 45 to 105 b.p.m.. Inherited insulin production rates can vary by a factor of 10, the low producers maybe predisposed to diabetes, and the high producers maybe predisposed to hyperinsulinism. The pepsin component of gastric acid can vary by a factor greater than 5,000 from one person to another. Even the shape of heart valves can vary drastically from person to person. [BI]

Additionally, the biochemistry within one individual is itself variant, hour by hour, day by day, month by month. It is well established that the reading of blood-pressure in a doctor's surgery may yield a value raised by the anxiety caused by the reading itself, along with fear of anticipation of a high reading. (An example of a self-fulfilling prophecy). The doctor should, but rarely does, also take a second blood-pressure reading via the other arm. They often mistakenly treat measurement *precision* as implying measurement *accuracy*. [BI]

Williams concluded that the diversity in our biochemistries had two main consequences. First, the huge range of chemicals within food will react differently with the diverse cocktails of internal chemistries from person to person. A foodstuff vital for one person can be almost a poison for another. Proof alone that one diet cannot fit all, and that simple nutritional advice normalised for the masses is almost meaningless. Second, that drugs also interact with differing human biochemistries in very different ways.

Additionally, not only has human biochemistry evolved great diversity, but our own biochemistry evolves during our life time. This evolution can be accelerated or at least heavily influenced by our nutrition. If we eat a diet that does not suit our biochemical needs, whether that is by virtue of excess, the wrong balance of food types, or simply poor quality foodstuffs, there will be an accumulative effect on our biochemistry. A principle example of this is of course type 2 diabetes, where the body cries out in complaint about the excess of carbohydrates entering the body over a prolonged period of time.

Ultimately, because our diversity makes illness diagnosis error-prone, and makes the effect of a drug vary from person to person, the avoidance of illness in the first place – prevention – is a much safer option than taking drugs after an illness has established itself.

Chapter Six

Taking control of our health

It is well established that the intake of Vitamins and Minerals staves off illnesses and strengthens the body. But matters of good nutrition, exercise and lifestyle factors are rarely addressed by physicians. These are 'soft' subjects, nice things to address, but deemed to bear too little relation to the serious matter of ill health. This is partly a result of the very narrow scope of medical education. The mechanics of the human body – its pathology – is the dominant focus. This induces an inflated sense of importance for bodily knowledge, elevated in its own sense of self-importance by the adoption of the obscure and often confusing medical terminology. The use of unfamiliar names for common body parts necessarily alienates medical staff from their patients. The body part feels alien to its owner by virtue of this naming convention. Medical practitioners seem to be reluctant to revert to more meaningful names. Why say patella when you can say kneecap?

Medical students only spend a tiny proportion of their many years of education training on the soft matters mentioned above. (Rarely ever touching on the even softer, but very real ability of the body to self-heal). The value of nutrition alone is seriously under-taught, yet it is one of the principle factors in your health.

Medical training focuses heavily on ill-health, rarely dealing with the prevention of ill-health, or with what can be learnt from those in good health. On reflection, it is a staggering reality that medical training seeks to offer us good health using examples of bad health as their guiding

45

force. The value of learning from the healthy amongst us seems to be almost entirely forgotten.

This is not entirely surprising in light of the obsession with symptomatic treatment (allopathic medicine), and the hijacking of medical education by the pharmaceutical industry, who furnish the drugs for that treatment. The educational spotlight is heavily focused on maladies and their obliteration, blinding us to the value that understanding of healthy people can bring us. Big Pharma (as I prefer to call them) has managed to leverage into the medical education curriculum a focus on the administration of drugs, establishing a pro-industry mind-set as early as possible. Much like 'Happy meals' at McDonalds establish a liking for the fast food experience in children. Catch children or medical students early enough and you may have them for life.

When those medical students who survive the arduous and lengthy medical training leave college, they encounter a world far removed from medical school. The sheer diversity of ailments and the people bringing these ailments to the doctor can be overwhelming. (Note that I use the words doctor and physician interchangeably, the former being the word more commonly used in the UK for the first stage port of call for medical care). In a sense, the doctor is starting from scratch, learning on the job how to deal with 'soft' matters such as human psychology and diversity for the first time. Alas, those that can endure the length, intensity and technical nature of medical education and training may well lack the skills required to deal with these very important soft matters. They are often thick-skinned, and highly focused on protecting their huge training investment. This often means a lack of empathy and a bias towards an academic, detached view of patients and the ailments that they bring with them.

The combination of these problems can lead to insensitive and poor handling of patients, and a drug initiated worsening of patient conditions. Ivan Illich used the term 'Iatrogenesis' to describe the damage that doctors can inflict on their patients. The word derives from the Greek Iatros, meaning physician, and genesis, meaning origin here.

He unfolds another, more subtle problem. A kind of meta-malpractice, where doctors hide behind the complexity and technical nature of modern treatments to distance themselves from blame. To quote Illich from his excellent book "The limits of medicine" [LM] :

"With the transformation of the doctor from an artisan exercising a skill on personally known individuals into a technician applying scientific rules to classes of patients, malpractice acquired an anonymous, almost respectable status ... The depersonalisation of diagnosis and therapy has changed malpractice from an ethical into a technical problem."

The more mechanical the care, the less personable it becomes, the more stressed the patient becomes, and the less likely they are to heal. This is no more so than in the anonymous environment of hospitals. Doctors and nurses wander around and through wards with a sense of the highest importance, relegating the bed bound patients to pawns in a game whose rules they do not really understand. Yet the medical staff are only there because of the patients, and should in general be subservient to them. Health care has been centralised, and mechanised, and I offer no apologies for quoting Illich again for his insightful commentary on this matter, describing here the patient experience :

"Now what he meets is the gaze of a biological accountant engaged in input/output calculations. His sickness is taken from him and turned into the raw material for an institutional enterprise."

The medical profession has divorced itself from the very people it is supposed to be serving. Just as with corporations (and indeed, note that private medical companies are often corporations), by growing huge, the focus of the medical profession becomes a self serving one. It feels a compunction to sustain its own existance and self-importance. And we are gradually conned into seeing the medical establishment as the only authority when it comes to our own personal health. Health care is centralised, where even the fringes – our local doctors – are caught up in the big scheme, heavily influenced by the pharmaceutical industry to push drugs as the only treatment. We even see our doctor when we have a cold.

Fundamentally, just like the doctors, we have lost our autonomy. We rarely question medical authority, nor when we do so do we do it with enough conviction. Surgery is becoming an ever more common treatment, yet the accompanying anaesthetics used are often brutally hard on the body, yet we are drawn into accepting them because it is offered from this position of unquestioned and unquestionable authority. We are so caught up with the acceptance of authority that they can administer surgery for even minor ailments without needing to offer any caveats.

It is worth pointing out that China regularly uses acupuncture and hypnosis in place of anaesthetics, and to good effect. It appears to be more effective, with less side effects, and a shorter hospital stay, with quicker and healthier recovery times. (Ogden, 2007).

The title of this chapter is intentionally ambiguous. They are indeed taking control of our health, but it should be us that take control of our health, and use the medical profession as a guide and aid – a supplement for matters beyond our abilities or resources.

The power of the medical profession and associated advisory bodies has corrupted them to the point where they actually seek to undermine many of our efforts at taking back control of our health. Alternative help for ailments, including nutrition and lifestyle matters are given this 'alternative' label in part to delegitimise them. It is true that our dissatisfaction with doctors has lead us to seek alternative medications, but we do so furtively, as if embarking on an illegal practice, unendorsed by big medicine.

By delegating control and responsibility for our health to others, we risk far too much. Illich tells of a revealing experiment carried out with the assistance of no less than 390 children. [LM] They asked a physician to determine which of these children should undergo a tonsillectomy, a procedure that removes the tonsils and tends to leave the patient with difficulty in swallowing for a few days, along with a sore throat for around two weeks. No less than 45% of the children were recommended to receive this treatment. Of those deemed OK, another physician was then asked for his opinion. Rather than give a clean bill of tonsil health to the vast majority of these children, he recommended a full 46% undergo the procedure. Remarkably, a similar percentage was given by a 3rd physician on the 'clear' remainder. Yet we have grown to trust the authority and decision making of medical staff without questioning because of the size and power of the medical profession. Or maybe I should call it the medical industry, for that, alas, is what it has become, having evolved to have the same kind of problems that corporations have acquired.

In his famous gem of a book, "The anatomy of an illness", [AI] Norman Cousins describes how he was diagnosed with a terminal and crippling illness. He soon found himself inside a depressing hospital, treated with aloofness by the medical staff, sliding towards death. With commendable bravado, and radical thinking, he signed himself out of the hospital and into a hotel, where he sat watching a stream of comedy films in sublime comfort. He recovered from his terminal condition, as all such good stories go, but because he broke the rules, the medical profession deemed his recovery to be spontaneous, dismissing his actions as incidental or anecdotal. Much better for the medical profession to retain power and control, even though they were handed a great new therapy on a plate (and indeed, laughter has been incorporated in enlightened medical establishments in the UK, Germany, India and other countries). To quote Cousins :

"No medication they could give their patients was as potent as the state of mind the patient brings to his or her illness"

But such alternative approaches involve no drugs, and hence no money for the big pharma, so they are unlikely to be embraced and therefore offered to patients. Yet doctors normally sign an oath – the Hippocratic oath – that implores them to explore alternatives before dismissing them as unworthy. But this ethical oath is long forgotten of course. ('Never do harm' is another key tenet in the oath, yet the administering of drugs with known side effects breaks this rule). It is also worth noting that both the mood of a doctor, or a clash of his personality with yours can generally adversely affect his ability to help you. In light of this, and the aforementioned shortcomings, if you want to use a doctor's diagnosis for your condition, it is better to get a 2nd and 3rd opinion if you can.

Unfortunately, this sorry picture is not complete yet. The greed of the pharmaceutical industry is relentless, it seems, happily pursuing corrupt and underhand practices to serve its 'needs'. A 2006 German led worldwide corruption survey found that pharmaceutical companies were amongst the worst [TT]. As mentioned earlier, they mislead newspaper readers with pseudo-scientific articles directing the reader to use their drugs. More devious than this, and much more widespread, is the fabrication of illnesses, which has become a serious and mushrooming concern.

It was recently realised that children represented a huge, mostly untapped market for medications. True, the drugs industry had made millions from drugs in the past such as Ritalin for children with ADHD (Attention Deficit Hyperactivity Disorder), in spite of the dangers of this strong drug. But now, they were looking to give anti-depressant drugs to children. Fortunately, these look like being withdrawn because of the ever real dangers of the suicidal tendency these can induce in some children.

Moving to women in mid life, Big Pharma is happy to diagnose as illnesses natural (but nevertheless very uncomfortable) events such as the menopause, and conjure up treatment to help these women cope better. Basically, any activity that can broaden and/or sustain their customer base is a candidate for exploitation. Market penetration it is called, and they care not about the morals of this expansion programme.

And what about the side effects? Can they really sell drugs that induce suicidal tendencies? Can they really play down or hide the negative aspects of their medications? They very much can and do, using a multi-pronged approach. First, they sponsor drug research, providing funding with strings attached to coerce favourable outcomes. It is hard to carry out impartial research when continued funding is dependent on the right results. However, the integrity of some researchers prevents them from manipulating results, so they choose to appease their funders by wording the research paper summary (abstract) in favour of the drug under test, playing down side effects or low efficacy. This can be almost as effective as a doctoring of results since the abstract is often the only part of a paper that gets read. Here they rely on a shortage of the resources (time and motivation) needed to find them out.

But they do not always avoid exposure. In 2010, GlaxoSmithKline (GSK) were found to be deliberately hiding the full extent of the heart attack risk for patients using their diabetic drug Avandia (see http://finance.senate.gov/press/Gpress/2010/prg022010a.pdf – it makes for enlightening reading). In order to suppress this serious risk, it appears that GSK employed intimidation against independent physicians, and used press releases to undermine an independent study that exposed the problem. GSK also found it appropriate to threaten a lawsuit against Dr John Buse, a diabetic specialist at the University of North Carolina who voiced concerns about Avandia. Lawsuits are often easier to win when you are a huge corporation. Additionally, it appears that the US FDA (Food and Drug Administration) were in cohorts, also playing down these serious side effects.

Not only do the pharmaceutical companies marginalise side effects of their drugs, but they poach government agencies as accomplices in their devious deeds. And governments actually compound this problem by allowing regulatory bodies, such as the FDA in the US, and the Medicines and Healthcare products Regulatory Agency (MHRA) in the UK, to charge drug companies for evaluating new drugs. [EN] The net effect being almost an overnight loss of impartiality.

That GSK might also want to resort to smear tactics, and intimidation, is more readily understood when you learn what they stood to lose if their drug was banned. In 2006 alone, global sales of Avandia was a staggering $3.4 Billion. Such an enormous revenue is too big to be jeopardised by a few studies. Way too much money to entertain feelings for the health of the diabetics prescribed the drug.

There are times when individual researchers, or whole research teams are hijacked by the drug companies, destroying their independence entirely. In 2009, a team of researchers led by Dr Scott Reuben was found guilty of faking the results of at least 21 pharmaceutical studies published in medical journals over a 13 year period. It was no small coincidence that two of the drugs, Bextra and Vioxx, that were reported as safe and effective, were produced by Pfizer and Merck, who paid Reuben for his work. When the fraud was revealed, these drug companies distanced themselves from him with typically clever public relations spin. For Pfizer, however, the illegal off-label promotion of Bextra was punished in 2009 with a fine and penalties amounting to $2.3 Billion, the largest criminal fine at that time.

It is worth repeating that in case you missed the full impact – the largest criminal fine by 2009 was incurred by a pharmaceutical company. And the victims of their crime were the many users of their 'approved' drug.

Howeverm, I must step aside for a moment. There is a strong, and very real danger here that my focus on the occasional misdeeds of *some* members of the pharmaceutical industry will cast them *all* in too negative a light. It is patently clear that they have delivered to many millions of patients across the world life and health saving medications. Likewise, the medical profession is equally a saviour to millions worldwide. But the majority of good work they do is seriously undermined by the aforementioned shortcomings that many people are simply not aware of.

It is of course understandable that drug manufacturers should seek to maximise sales, especially if the scale of these sales is enormous. To bring a drug to market can take many years, and hundreds of millions of dollars, so demanding is the route imposed upon them. In addition, many drugs fall by the wayside, failing to reach the market. When a drug finally receives approval, the return on the investment is partly achieved by volume of sales. But the key driver of profit is the manufacturing to retail cost markup. And this can be staggeringly high at times.

'Big Pharma' also take the meta step of owning or funding many of the pharmaceutical journals, allowing them to exercise some control over which papers are selected, and push towards drug-favourable presentation of results. This is akin to the hijacking of newspapers of course. The Journal of the American Medical Association (JAMA) probably could not exist without drug funding. And funding is also used to influence medical organisations, damaging their independence. The American Diabetic Association (ADA) is so dependent on industry funding that it rarely declares any foods as bad for diabetics. This, of course, can result in a damaging effect on the many millions of diabetic sufferers that assume that they are given impartial and sensible advice from such advisory bodies.

On a smaller scale, but more immediately telling to the masses, physicians are often bombarded by drug companies with gifts, education (indoctrination) and funding solely for the promotion and hence prescribing of their drugs. Here in the UK, a significant proportion of the potential income for a doctor is in the form of prescription bonuses. Each time the doctor enrols another patient in a course of one of a number of selected medications, he is rewarded. This makes independence and impartiality very hard to maintain. The sad matter is that it is not the drug industry making the payments directly to the doctors – they have managed to convince governments to do so on their behalf. They rely on the authority of the government to promote their products.

Chapter Seven
Taking control of our food

Although I have mentioned nutrition briefly so far, it will play a large role in this book, much as it does in your own welfare. It is almost the case of *"Garbage in, garbage out"*. But before I go any further, it must be pointed out that nutrition – the food that we eat – is a massively complex subject. The vast quantity and diversity of chemicals in food interacts with the vast quantity and diversity of chemicals in humans. When complexity meets a diversity of complexities, how can we be sure of the value of any universal message? We literally cannot know what the effect of eating a head of raw broccoli will have on us. I love eating all sorts of nuts and legumes, but some unfortunate people can suffer fast onset anaphylactic shock after eating as little as one peanut, or a sprinkling of sesame seeds.

You are aware already of the potential consequences of omitting one chemical – Vitamin A – from the diet, so can see how important food is to our health. Big industry – and in particular Big foood – has a dominant and growing involvement in what we eat, and in line with the general theme of the book so far, you will probably guess that they often put their financial security and growth ahead of food quality. This is a sad reality, but it is the *degree* to which industry derails our nutritional health that is the saddest matter. Yet they claim innocence, of course. In simple terms, the food industry places its profit before your health. It can readily do so because the aforementioned complexity of nutrition acts as a smokescreen. And also because the majorit of people have a relatively low levels of nutritional understanding.

It is a sad failing of the educational system that you are much more likely to be informed about the history of your country in the 20th century than you are about what food is good for you in the 21st century. Not only are we generally ill-informed, but we are also easily fooled, often in subtle ways. For example, it is a common practice for supermarkets to offer fruit and vegetables that are colourful and well formed. The visual aesthetics rarely correlate, however, with the nutritional value. A head of broccoli grown rapidly using chemicals in a greenhouse may actually look more perfect than one grown organically in rich soil, yet will often contain less vitamins and minerals.

One of the most profitable routes the food industry takes is in the manufacturing of food. They transfer the production line concept of mass market consumer goods to the manufacture of food stuffs. With an endless supply of fast and reliably grown grains as the staple component, a whole plethora of processed foods such as cereals, cakes and biscuits can literally be manufactured. More often than not, the grains are stripped of many nutrients and fibre in order to maximise the taste of the end product. Plant oils are used as the fat component of the products to ensure good taste, with fruit sugars increasingly used as the sweetener.

This also serves to illustrate a concerted drive away from animal products. This is not for any ethical reasons but simply for financial and logistical ones. It is much simpler to harvest sunflower seeds as the fat ingredient in a biscuit than it is to grow and nurture cows, milk them, and convert the milk into butter. This is evident in the large amount of floor space that is given to grain and grain-based products than to animal products. It is no small coincidence that the latter are slower and more labour intensive to produce. Time consuming, hard to manage processes, such as the rearing and slaughtering of livestock is best minimised if profit is your focus. To reinforce the consumption of grain-based products, animal products have been given a bad name. The food industry promotes high profit lines, and demotes low profit lines.

But in a global sense, there is a much bigger driving force behind the focus on grains. The world is fundamentally overpopulated, and has been for decades. At the time of writing, the population is close to 7 billion, a rise of nearly a billion in the last decade alone. It may come as a surprise to you to know that the world population was only 2.5 billion as recently as 1950. For a large percentage of the world population, especially India and China, animal products are simply a luxury. It is much more efficient to grow grains to feed these vast numbers. Crudely put, food quantity rather than quality becomes the focus. For around 3 billion people, rice (a grass seed) is the staple of their diet. Whilst it is understandable for many to subsist on grains, I will explore the claim that it is healthier to consume animal products. Yet the drive to make grains as a staple for all is not constrained to these large numbers of poor people. Those who can afford to eat animal products often stop doing so, made to believe by industry that it is better for their health to avoid them.

Before I leave the influence of 'Big Food', I will cover some more detailed examples of their malpractices. No better place to start than with margarine, the so-called 'healthy' alternative to butter. Except, of course, that it is not. Margarine is the generic name for butter substitutes. In general, a vegetable oil is bleached, dyed, flavoured and enriched to resemble butter. The more processed a product, the less healthy it is likely to be for us. Imagine a new line in margarines – 'pure, simple and unadulterated'. But who would buy a grey, tasteless hard oil? 'Sales would plummet', to quote from Monty Python's Flying Circus.

Compare and contrast with pure, unadulterated and delicious butter made in a farm from certified raw milk. In 1993, a Harvard Nurses study of over 80,000 women found that those eating 4-6 teaspoons of margarine daily were 66% more likely to suffer with heart disease than those eating the same amount of butter. One of those who recognised the value of quality butter said :

"We buttered everything from broccoli to brownies, and would have buttered butter itself if it were not for the problems of traction presented by the butter-butter interface."

Proctor and Gamble spent 30 years seeking approval for Olestra [FP] as a nutritional fat substitute. Olestra tastes like fat, but essentially passes through the body, seemingly therefore a boon for dieters. But it was this unhindered passage of Olestra that caused the delay in approval, since it resulted in loose stools. The fat most familiar to the human body is triglyceride – literally a glycerol backbone with 3 fat linkage sites. Olestra uses sucrose as a backbone. The body fails to absorb Olestra because its structure is too large – it has 8 fat linkage sites. Not long after hitting the market, the FDA received thousands of complaints, forcing Proctor and Gamble to add a warning to the product label. It would not surprise you to learn that subsequent intense lobbying saw this warning removed from the packaging. Why? Because it cost \$500 million to bring to the market, and the warning was affecting sales. In essence, Olestra is a non-food, damaging to your body, yet Proctor and Gamble spent decades fighting the Food and Drug Administration and common sense to force it upon us as something worthy of eating.

Many foods are promoted as super-foods, vital to health. And, indeed, many do seem to deserve this accolade. However, most of us do not have the resources to determine how true these claims are, except to suck it and see. The difficulty there, however, is that we cannot separate the effect of the food from the many other influences on our health, not least our expectation that the food is going to be good for us. Can we measure the extent and effectiveness of blueberries as an anti-oxidant food? Do we indeed need to curb the effects of oxidation within the body? There is indeed some doubt on this matter.

In 1994, the US Congress worryingly passed the 'Dietary supplement health and education act', almost certainly as the result of industry lobbying. It allowed dietary supplements to be free from regulation, requiring only that they be declared as safe to consume. The manufacturer did not have to prove efficacy and safety of their product – it was up to the FDA to disprove. With the sheer volume of products on the market, this mechanism was never going to reliably protect the public from bad products. Certainly not in an appropriately timely manner.

By no small coincidence, a company called Mannatech started selling 'Glyconutrients' to a vulnerable public in the very same year. Glyconutrients are 8 purportedly essential sugars that we apparently rarely encounter in our diet. With sufficient scientific plausibility to fool the public, but with no actual supporting science, Mannatech managed to achieve annual sales of $400 million in 2007, the same year in which the Glycobiology Journal eventually exposed their activity as a scam. These sugars were not vital to health. Bizarrely, the Mannatech web site even admitted that their product did not treat or cure disease. Contrary, however, to the claims made by the large sales force selling glyconutrients to an unsuspecting and vulnerable public. We can be sold a product with no proven health value simply because industry can get away with it.

Chapter Eight
Food advice for the masses

Before I explore some aspects of historical UK and US nutritional advice, it is worth jumping the gun a little to give an example of the consequence of some of the simple, enduring and often misleading advice we are given. To quote Marion Nestle [FP] :

> *"Fat is fattening, it contains more than twice the calorific value of equal amounts of carbs or protein"*

This is assumed to be so self evident that Nestle sees no need to explain the logic behind this 'fact'. First, she fails to define what is meant by 'amounts'. Is she referring to volume or weight? Are the carbs in question raw, or steamed, or boiled or grilled? But the main problem here is a failure to look beyond the foods themselves and observe the interaction of these food types with the human digestive tract.

Fats, carbohydrates and proteins are all processed very differently from each other. They are also processed differently from hour to hour and day to day as our bodily needs vary. And we rarely eat these food types in isolation – different combinations of these foods results in different assimilations. But the key fact that is overlooked by Nestle and many others is that our stomachs are much more keenly sensitive to the calorific value of food than its volume or weight. Just as the digestive system is aware that full fat cheese is nutrient dense, and thereby makes us fuller more readily, it will likewise keep us hungry when we have eaten a dozen sticks of celery. Fat may be more nutrient dense than carbohydrate or protein, but our bodies are not deceived by such matters.

By the way, we have Wilbur Atwater to blame for the concept of the calorie. He determined the calorific value of food by burning it in a calorimeter, measuring the heat released. That this was quite different from how the human body 'burnt' food did not appear to be a problem to him.

The food advice history I cover here is principally that which relates to the balance of food types we consume as opposed to the nutritional benefits of individual foods. I will start way back in 1863, with William Banting, an English undertaker who was despairing at his corpulence. Whilst robust figures were deemed favourable at the time, his was somewhat too large. He was obese, and struggled to lose weight until he adopted a diet low in easily digested carbohydrates on the advice of Dr. William Harvey. This particular diet had been the subject of diabetic management lectures Harvey had attended in Paris. He suspected that the weight loss diabetics incurred on the diet could transfer safely to non-diabetics like Banting.

So successful was the diet that it moved Banting to write a booklet entitled 'Letter on Corpulence, Addressed to the public', where he detailed the many and varied failed methods he had tried in order to lose weight. He explained that it was only when he adopted a diet whose principle feature was an omission of starches and sugars – the fast acting carbohydrates – that he reliably lost weight. Whilst the booklet was well received by those who tried the diet, it was rejected by the medical community. Banting became ridiculed for his advice, and rumours were spread that the diet was damaging his health. Note that in the 19th Century, heart-disease was at very low levels in spite of the large amount of meat and fat eaten. TT

The problem here was a combination of the anecdote of a single person and a radical message. The lack of weight in the message that an unspecialised person provided, no matter how valid, stood no chance against the inertia of nutritional understanding at the time. By the same token that *misinformation* repeated loud enough and often enough by people in positions of authority can become believed and accepted, *valid information* voiced once by an individual is rejected if it is deemed too implausible.

The American Francis Gano Benedict explored rest, exercise and diet in over 500 experiments from 1895 to 1906. From 1907 to 1936 he worked in the Boston Nutrition Laboratory, developing basal metabolism measurement devices. In 1917, he studied the effect of a traditional low-calorie diet on metabolism. The tests involved a two stage diet. His subjects were fed a 1400 calorie diet for a few weeks, followed by a 2100 calorie diet, both below their normal 2500 calorie daily intake. The diet was relatively 'balanced', with sizeable amounts of carbohydrates.

During the first period, all the participants complained of a constant, gnawing hunger. Thoughts of food were dominant. They were cold, weak and tired. Their bodies had responded to the low calorie diet by a lowering of metabolism. The most telling aspect though was the consequences of the move to 2100 calories, where the lowered metabolic level and its deleterious effects persisted. The additional calories were not used to raise metabolism, but were stored as fat.

The experiment did not finish when the diet ended – the subjects were monitored when subsequently given unlimited food. They were found to have capacious appetites, averaging an 8 lb gain over their pre-diet weight. The results were published in "Human vitality and efficiency under a prolonged restricted diet". This study confirmed what most people suspected – restricting calories was not in itself the remedy to sustained weight loss. However, a low-calorie diet persisted as the recommended route for obese people until the 1950's.

In the 1920's, Sir John Boyd was a nutritional adviser to the UK government. In order to allay problems of ill health in poor children, he recommended that their diet be supplemented by milk. This had the desired effect, partly because of the quality of full-fat milk at the time (more on this matter later).

In the same flavour, from the 1930's to the 1950's, the UK government recommended the following dietary changes :

- 80% more milk
- 55% more eggs
- 40% more butter
- 30% more meat

Such recommendations are clearly at odds with current dietary advice. However, the advice was not only heeded, but a general reduction of disease rates followed.

In the 1940's in the US, the Journal of the American Medical Association (JAMA) published research by Alfred Pennington. Hired by the medical department of E. I. DuPont, he had taken the idea from Banting's booklet and tested it scientifically. He had moved the idea from anecdote to the scientific method, testing the efficacy of a diet unrestricted in calories, but restricted in carbohydrates on a group of obese subjects. Gone were the obsessive hunger pangs – the subjects coped comfortably on a diet restricted in calories, but also in carbohydrates. The higher fat levels used as energy in such a diet appeared to satiate the appetites of the subjects much longer.

Legitimising his findings in a well respected journal should have been enough for the low-carbohydrate approach to dieting to defeat the low-calorie method. Alas, the diet was criticised as dangerous to health. It was not deemed important that the 20 subjects of the diet lost an average of 22 lbs each over a period of three and a half months. That they did so without feeling hungry, in spite of being on a low-calorie diet, was also lost on the critics.

Here again the power of strong voices are shown to trample over profoundly valuable findings. It is another example of a minority of humans suppressing a gain for the many, on arbitrary, subjective grounds. This oppression quashed what should have been a great opportunity for further research – exactly why were obese people able to lose weight and yet not feel hungry in the process? This was contrary to intuition and begged for a deeper investigation. But it appears that it was too taboo for anyone to be prepared for such an undertaking.

At the Royal Society of Medicine in London in 1950, Sir Charles Dodds carried out research on metabolism that added a further spanner to the works. It did not seek to confirm or refute the efficacy of a low-carbohydrate diet, but instead explored the effect of human metabolic variations on the assimilation of food. The subjects for the experiment he carried out fell into two categories. Group one consisted of those whose weight was historically known to remain essentially constant regardless of exercise and food consumption. Group two consisted of those unfortunate people who tended to put on weight easily.

He over fed each group to see the effect. Not just over fed, but sometimes as much as 3 times their normal calorific intakes. Those with stable weights barely put on any weight, whereas the unstable weight group laid on the pounds. The inevitable conclusion was that the stable weight group had a highly flexible metabolism that helped to normalise their weight. They literally burned off the extra food. However, the metabolism of those in the other group barely changed during the experiment, so that a lot of the extra food was stored as fat.

The stark and very simple conclusion here is that one diet does not fit all. And there is also the very sad reality that there are likely to be many people who literally have to starve themselves to stay at a stable weight. Life can be very much unfair – for those with a static metabolism, weight loss on any kind of low-calorie diet was ultimately going to be a painful, ineffective activity.

Another twist to dietary advice came in the 1950's when big industry started pushing vegetable oils. One of the casualties was coconut oil, which was the target of a smear campaign that marginalised this superb food for decades. It was deemed too big a competition to corn and soy oils that were earmarked as large money earners for Big Food. (Read more about the extent of this brutally unfair treatment here : www.thaifoodandtravel.com/features/cocgood.html). Yet coconuts are a natural source of food, and form a staple part of the diet of many people. They are the richest source of medium chain fatty acids. Coconut oil goes directly to the liver as fuel, yet does not raise blood sugar levels. A fast fuel without side-effects, and hence ideal for those with poor digestion.

It additionally aids calcium and magnesium absorption, stimulates metabolism, and strengthens the immune system. As if this was not enough, coconut oil is also anti-fungal, anti-bacterial and anti-viral. Yet it is labelled as unhealthy.

This damning of alternatives used by big industry to promote vegetable oil also extended to saturated fat, as found in many animal products. And this was an easy target. Whilst the fat on meat was tasty, it was all too easy to relate dietary-fat to body-fat. Saturated fat was also indicted in the clogging of arteries. In spite of the fact that research did not back up these two matters, a very belligerent, highly persuasive physiologist named Ancel Keys picked up on the 'fat is bad' concept and pushed the US government to advise US citizens to reduce their fat intake.

But the research at the time did not show a correlation between body fat and dietary fat intake, nor a correlation between fat consumption and cardiovascular diseases (CVD). For ten years, Keys was rejected by both government and their nutritional advisers. [DD] But in addition to being persuasive, Keys was also stubborn, and submitted a paper in 1953 entitled 'Atherosclerosis, a problem in newer public health'. Keys manipulated the data in this report to enforce his beliefs, cherry picking just 6 countries out of 22 for which research had looked at the relation between saturated fat consumption and cardiovascular-disease. [DD] However, Keys was still not accepted by the US government. They were, however, being worn down by his persistence.

Four years later, Jacob Yerushalmy Ph.D., founder of the University of California at Berkeley Bio-Statistics graduate program reported that there was no correlation between saturated fat consumption and CVD when the statistics from all 22 countries were taken into account, confirming the manipulation that Keys resorted to in order to push his message. Nutritionist John Yudkin also sought to counter the anti-fat dogma that Keys was promoting by himself advocating a low-carbohydrate diet.

In 1956, Professor Alan Kekwick and Dr. G. L. S. Pawan at Middlesex Hospital in London researched the efficacy of Banting's diet. They were successful, and summarised their findings very neatly :

"The composition of the diet can alter the expenditure of calories in obese persons, increasing it when fat and proteins are given and decreasing it when carbohydrates are given"

The obese participants in their research were found to lose weight on a 2,600 calorie diet if that diet were high in fat. A diet lower in fat would yield weight loss only if the calorie level was reduced.

Meanwhile, observations such as in Charleston, USA were being ignored as anecdotal. African Americans in that city were malnourished on low-calorie, high-carbohydrate diets yet were becoming obese. This failure to investigate findings that countered conventional wisdom is a common failing of the scientific, medical and nutrition communities. Meanwhile, in 1960, the growing understanding of the combined failure of low-calorie diets and the success of low-carbohydrate diets was shunted aside when Keys produced a version of his anti-fat report that was at last accepted by the US government. It appears that he survived rejection by omitting references. He relied on common sense to push his ideas across. And an edition of Time magazine hailed him as a hero of the times.

As mentioned earlier, as soon as governments adopt an idea, it is likely to stay unchanged for a long time, regardless of any contrary information. Continuity of communication so often takes precedence over accuracy. A baseline for future nutritional advice was being established – on faulty evidence. The power of the message, rather than its validity proved to be key. It was easy to push the message because common sense reinforced it – how easy it is to mistakenly equate dietary fat with body fat.

Keys followed up in 1970 with the Seven Countries study that explored the link between saturated-fat intake and heart attacks. Except that, true to form, he fudged the statistical observations. His correlation did not exist for three of the seven countries. Three out of seven is of course a dangerously high level to ignore, undermining the value of his claims. But the US government readily accepted research that reinforced the direction they had chosen, even if the original basis for this choice was itself based on flawed research.

However, there was a growing unrest with many concerning this blight on fat, and in particular the innocent status that carbohydrates were acquiring, in spite of Kekwick and Pawan's findings. One man sought to fight back against the system, revitalising Banting's diet. His surname is very famous of course, and has become the generic name for low-carbohydrate diets. Dr. Robert Atkins made effective dieting accessible to the masses in his extremely popular 'The Atkins diet' book. In the 1970's, millions adopted his version of the Banting diet, and many not only lost weight but stayed on the diet as a lifestyle choice.

But the medical and nutritional experts at the time were still very unhappy about any diet that recommended high fat intake. The government's adoption of a low-fat stance was already having wide-spread influence. Sadly, Atkins chose to add an emotional tone to his book, taking an opportunity to have a dig at those who criticised fat. This was the achilles heel of his book, causing critics to take umbrage, slating the book as unscientific and as promoting eating practices dangerous to health. Once again, the benefits of a low-carbohydrate diet were lost under the weight of a smear campaign.

1977 was to be a landmark year in this saga. Against the advice of both the scientific community and the American Medical Association (AMA), Congress made the low-fat diet government policy the 'Dietary goal'. Hard as it is to believe in the 21st century, the idea of a low-fat diet was actually very badly received by the people and nutritional advisers. But the most alarming facet of this new goal was that *low-fat diets had not been tested.* Advice for the whole US population had not even been validated. Glib statements that fat was higher in calories than carbohydrates went unquestioned. The strength of the message blinded the listeners to its false foundations.

In the 1980's, the focus had moved on to the dangers of cholesterol. Once again, Time magazine latched onto this new villain of health, giving it the front page. The attack on fat had taken a new twist – it was claimed now that the consumption of too much saturated-fat raised cholesterol levels, increasing the risk of heart-disease. By 1987, the US National Institute of Health (NIH) decreed that physicians should put patients on cholesterol lowering drugs if their cholesterol levels were greater than 200 mg/dl. And here you see Big Pharma revealing its ugly head again. The 'fat is bad' mantra was being exploited for money making purposes by the drug industry. I will speak more on this later.

The efficacy of the recommended low-fat diet was eventually subject to scientific scrutiny in a series of 6 medium sized studies from 1988 to 1994. [DD] They failed to show the health benefits of a low-fat diet, so the results were each deemed to be 'single case' exceptions. Mad though this is, when a message such as the low-fat mantra has accumulated enough momentum, it takes a disproportionate amount of effort to derail it. There are parallels here with the scientific community, holding onto long held theories with an iron grip, in spite of an accumulation of contradictory evidence. In both cases, there is too much to be lost to give up without a fight. A fight against reason in many cases.

In the 1990's, there was a growing awareness of the dangers of refined carbohydrates, but even this was diffused by a clever little sidestep. Rather than incur any blight on the high revenue earning refined carbohydrates market, Big Food pushed the focus to the fibre that refined carbohydrates lacked. It was claimed that fibre added to your diet was seen as the boost to health all should benefit from. As already discussed, this technique of deflection was one also used by many politicians. And rightly so, if your aims are not honourable, since it is a very effective trick to use. [DD]

In spite of the dangers of refined carbohydrates, claims to good health on processed food packaging was actually endorsed by the American Heart Association (AHA) in 1993. [FP] In order to increase its funding, the AHA accepted initial and annual fees from Big Food for product endorsements, often on foods high in sugar. The health of the masses became very much a secondary issue as far as industry and advisory bodies were concerned.

Meanwhile, the 'dangers' of saturated-fat were again refuted by research. A study in 1997 appearing in JAMA showed stroke rates were lower in 832 men on a high saturated-fat diet. A 2004 Harvard University study of heart disease patients revealed that the more fat they ate, the less likely their conditions would deteriorate. A 2009 Women's Health Initiative $725 million study into the effect of a low-fat, low-saturated-fat diet on cardiovascular-health revealed no benefits. But these findings were incapable of dislodging the entrenched evil status that fat had acquired.

Over the past few decades, guidance on the balance of foods to eat for good health has been summarised by the FSA 'Eat Well' diagram in the UK and the 'Food Pyramid' in the US. Of course, they reflect the

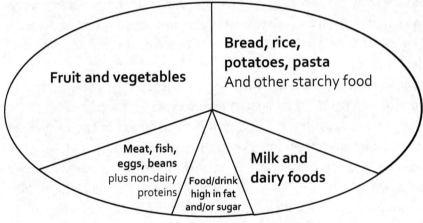

Figure 1 : The UK FSA Eat Well plate

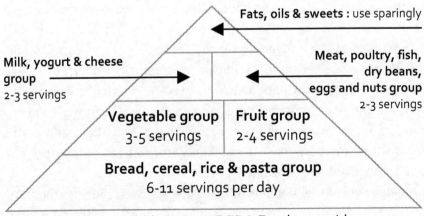

Figure 2 : The 1992 US FDA Food pyramid

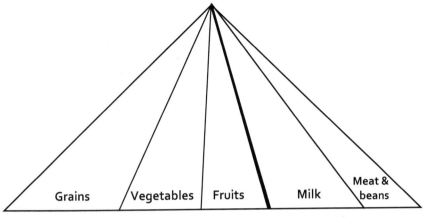

Figure 3 : The 2005 US FDA Food Pyramid

anti-fat and pro-carbohydrate dogmas. Grain based products occupy the largest component of their recommended diets, and 'nasty' oils and fats the lowest. Although the diagrams are meant to advise us on the proportions of foods we should eat for a healthy diet, they are badly organised and misleading. Until the 2005 version of the Food Pyramid revision, both displayed sugary foods as a result of pressure from the food industry. FP

Both the current Eat Well plate and the 1992 Food Pyramid grouped sugars and fats into a separate category, stigmatising fat further in the process. But separating out these 'demons' confuses of course, since fat and sugar is found in varying degrees in most foods. Dose this mean that avocados are bad to eat because they contain high fat levels? And what about butter and cheese in the dairy category? The message to the public is simply misleading.

Each of these diagrams succumbs to excessive simplicity. The bolt-on fats and sugars category is even an admission that simple is not meaningful enough, unable to even start to address the full facts. For example, as mentioned before, no indication is given as to what constitutes a portion of fruit or vegetables, and what balance between fruits and vegetables should be struck.

The 1992 food pyramid at least attempts to recommend portions of each food category per day, but is it really prudent advice to suggest as many as 11 portions of carbohydrates per day in light of what has been revealed about them? The idea of the Eat Well plate segment sizes, and the sizes and elevation in the 1992 Food Pyramid give a sense of food balance recommended. Even if the proportions are misguided (they really do hate us to eat meat and poultry), the 2005 Food Pyramid completely gives up on the pyramid concept, yet still uses the pyramid shape, but to no effect whatsoever. It has an additional flaw that reveals a lot about the government attitude towards dietary fat. Notice that the line between the Fruit and Milk triangles is thicker than the other lines? It is in fact an additional triangle, but totally lacking a label, and hence readily overlooked. This is the 'Oils' column.

Although I have essentially covered only one aspect of nutrition in this very brief history, barely scratching the surface of this vast subject, the drive to demonise fat has single handedly damaged the lives of millions of people. The anti-fat message was based on flawed reporting to government, and capitalised on by the food industry as a mechanism for selling us the high profit refined carbohydrates that are the real demon. But this is only part of the Big Food story. It is time now to step back to the start of the food chain, and see where Big Chemistry also gets to play a part in damaging our health.

Chapter Nine

From the soil beneath our feet

The importance of the very soil under our feet is often overlooked. Most of the land and air based food chain starts there, yet we tend to see soil as little more than a dirty brown substance. The end product of the activity of a raft of life-forms, a good soil is of course a prime growing medium for plant life. Bacteria and the protozoa that eat the bacteria are principle participants of soil metabolism. Fungi break down organic matter (such as manure and leaves that mulch down into the soil), and nematodes (mostly worms) recycle nutrients and keep some plant attacking species at bay. As importantly, they aerate the soil, which also improves drainage. Their excretions are a vital source of plant food, accessed by roots. Plants and the animals that eat them represent a large proportion of the food we eat.

Unknown to most people, rocks form a vital part of soil fertility. It leaches a wealth of minerals into the soil food chain. These minerals eventually make their way into plants via their roots. Another source of minerals is the aforementioned organic matter that drops onto the soil from above. Sometimes, the soil mineral balance gets out of kilter, damaging not only the plant life but also the animals that eat these plants. Yet soil mineral profiling is a relatively simple test, and rapid results can be achieved by rebalancing with mineral additives.

Every decade from 1940 to 1991, Dr. R. A. McCame and E. M. Widdowson published the nutrient content of popular foods. Over this half century, they noticed a significant decline in mineral content. [ww] For example, the overall nutritional value of a tomato in 1940 was equivalent to ten tomatoes in 1991. Selenium, calcium, iron, magnesium, zinc and copper levels in foods are now so low that most people fail to consume a healthy amount. There is evidence that indicates that low dietary mineral levels are at least part cause of many illnesses and diseases such as dyslexia and aspergers syndrome, along with high levels of teenage violence and anti-social behaviour (although all of these are highly likely to be multi-factorial behaviours). [ww] Young offenders were often found to be deficient in selenium, magnesium and zinc. When treated with supplements for 9 months, offence levels and behaviour improved. [ww]

The quality of the soil is of course fundamental to the quality of the food that derives from it. This can hardly be overstated, yet is readily overlooked. Soil quality is hardly an inspiring matter, yet it is a critical one. In light of this importance, it is deeply worrying that the vast quantity of food production, and hence soil management, is now controlled by big industry. Big Food as I call them. And as you are now acutely aware, revenue and profit are often more important to Big Food than our health.

One of the key soil components that affects the growth of plants is nitrogen. In a drive to accelerate plant growth, farmers were coaxed into using nitrogen fertilisers. This is now, sadly, common practice, but the rapid growth comes at a price. Structurally, the plants are weakened, prone to the effects of wind and driving rain. They are also more vulnerable to disease. There is a parallel here with the side-effects of drugs. In both cases, the side-effects should be seen as signals that the path being taken is the wrong one – both for the plant and the consumers of the plant in this case.

Additional chemicals are then required to defend against the increased vulnerability to disease that rapid plant growth creates, and also to kill the weeds that can grow around these prolific but frail plants. The problem does not stop there, however, because the animals that eat the plants are then administered anti-biotics to protect them from the effect of the unexpected and certainly unwanted chemicals they now consume. A vicious cycle has erupted once again, all in the name of higher yields to fuel industry's insatiable appetite for profit.

Because the cost of the application of chemicals is actually very high, governments subsidise their use. Governments in effect pay to introduce toxins into the food chain so that industry can get rich. Without the subsidy, these chemicals would be prohibitively expensive, and there would be less riches to be had! This sorry state of affairs is likely to be entrenched because the chemical industry now stands to lose a lot if organic farming were to move beyond its fringe position. Not only is the soil heavily loaded with chemicals, but the delicate combination of micro-organisms is badly damaged, and the vital pockets of air create by worms are lost, making drainage poor. Many chemically treated soils become almost inert. [ww]

Organic farming is based on methods that have been tried and tested for centuries. The cornerstone to their approach is the avoidance of chemicals. But there are more subtle aspects to good organic farming that separate it from its chemical-dependant counterpart. Historically, livestock roamed and fed on fields that were stocked with hundreds of plant types. A mix of old fashioned grasses and clover results in a greater variety of root depth, and hence optimal extraction of the nutrients found at various levels within the soil. A poor mix of grasses, as often happens today, can result in poor soil nutrient extraction leading to grazing animal developmental problems, such as tuberculosis in cattle. [ww] If the right mineral and vitamin balance is achieved in the soil, and a wide range of grasses are deployed to maximise nutrient extraction, then grazing animals will grow to be strong and healthy, and yield the healthiest meats and dairy for human consumption. Beef from healthy cows, for example, contains higher levels of Conjugated Linoleic Acid (CLA), Eicosapentaenoic Acid (EPA) and Dososahexaenoic Acid (DHA), all of which are vital for good health. [ww]

But Big Food is generally more interested in rapid yield than in quality. The drive for more at lower costs has moved cows away from the fields to live a mostly enclosed, grain fed life. The encampment in catttle 'sheds' both physically and emotionally cripples these poor animals. Grains are not only easier and cheaper to use as food stock, but they are also favoured since they fatten cows faster than grass does. Cows, however, are ruminants, so named after their first stomach, the ruman, which is used to break down grass. They have not really evolved to eat grains, and often suffer inflammation of the ruman as a consequence. But they fatten faster, so Big Food is happy.

As a little aside here, I have to admit to being puzzled that cows are powerful beasts, yet happily subsist on just grasses (much as pandas live principally on bamboo). We humans, a much weaker species, need a food profile that has a fairly close match to our bodily profile – dietary proteins and fats are vital to our health. We have evolved this way, but in principle, I guess we could eventually evolve to manufacture our all own fats and proteins as cows do, given enough time of course.

Big Food was not content with rapid cow-fattening of course, and eventually introduced fast-growing, high milk-yielding cows such as the Holstein in placed of long established stock. Here in the UK, quality breeds such as the Hereford and Sussex are now in decline as a result. Quantity usurps quality yet again. Milk yields in the UK rose from around 3,500 litres per cow per year in the 1960's to current levels of around 10,000 litres.

But the subject of milk quality is a large and pervasive one. Older breeds of cattle produce milk with high A2 beta casein protein levels. This protein has been shown by many studies to be linked with a *reduction* in health risks (see www.betacasein.org). Human breast milk, for example, contains A2 beta casein protein. Conversely, modern high yield breeds produce milk with high A1 beta casein protein levels. A1 beta casein is harder to digest for humans.

The modern higher yielding cows are given additional anti-biotics because their immense udders are more prone to mastitis. The sheer weight of their lactic cargo also causes hind leg damage, often leading to premature death. Synthetic growth hormones fed to the cows also ends up in their milk, a source of ill health for human consumers (see 'Bovine somatotropinon' on Wikipedia). This is a sorry state of affairs we find ourselves in, all a simple consequence of industrial greed.

Big Food was not content with 'just' this sacrifice of quality and health for higher profits, and exacerbated the problem further by replacing the very healthy, but slow production of raw milk from quality cows with high volume, lower quality milk that is then damaged by pasteurisation.

Part of the drive to pasteurise milk was most likely to eradicate a collection of chemicals that appeared in the milk as a result of the aforementioned problems. But it was also in part because of increased shelf life. Pasteurisation allows Big Food to cover its tracks and maximise sales by avoiding the likelihood of milk going sour, or causing ill-health. The reduced tendency to sour is a hallmark of a more inert, and hence less healthy product. Yet well run small farms here in the UK and in the US can and do produce raw milk with safely low bacterial levels.

Pasteurisation involves heating milk to high temperatures in order to kill a large proportion of potentially dangerous bacteria. However, 90% of the enzymes in the milk are also destroyed, and some of these are required for the proper digestion of the milk! There appears to be evidence (www.realmilk.com/safety-raw-milk.html) that lactose intolerance is more a consequence of the pasteurisation process than an inherent feature of cow's milk. (One writer for that web site reported that when he started drinking certified raw milk, not only did it alleviate the mucus and digestion problems he had, but it also started reversing the arthritic condition he had in his foot). The depletion of enzymes in the milk may well serve to reduce the assimilation of calcium within it. Not only that, but pasteurisation also damages the milk proteins, and depletes the calcium, phosphorous and iodine levels as well. [HY]

After pasteurisation, the milk is placed in a centrifuge, separating out the fat and leaving behind skimmed milk, which is heat treated again. Some of the separated fat is added back to make full-fat or semi-skimmed milk. For most supermarket milk, the fat undergoes one final process before this recombination. This process is called homogenisation.

To understand why even further degradation of a fine natural product was introduced, you have to look at the motives of the Supermarkets who instigated it. Not only did they seek low-bacteria safety assurances for their supplied milk, and a long shelf life, they also looked for a way to stop the cream rising up to the top and clogging the pouring process. They wanted the milk to look uniform – for the fat to be evenly distributed throughout the milk. Homogenisation literally means a process to achieve a homogenous or uniform appearance. The supermarkets obsessed more about visual and pouring matters than the taste or quality of the milk. For these aesthetic matters, they condemned the majority of us to drink milk that had undergone not one, but two stages of degradation.

This drive to create a uniform appearance was made at a great cost to its quality. The homogenisation process reduces the fat globules to a uniformly small size, where the globule-wall to contained-fat ratio is massively increased. Too much whey and casein and too little fat. The assimilation of the fat is reduced by the globule size. A lower fat content in milk (especially the essentially fat-free skimmed milk) also means a lower uptake of the fat soluble Vitamins A, D and K. Synthetic vitamins are actually added to the milk in an attempt to compensate for this degrading nature of this process, but note here that synthetic vitamin D actually interferes with the uptake of calcium. Better to have natural vitamins than added ones.

Stepping right back now, to a time decades ago when many humans were involved in daily hard physical work, we can see the multifactorial affect on health that time has brought. The energy needs of a labourer would likely be 1.5 to 2 times that of an office worker – maybe 4,000 to 5,000 calories versus around 2,500 calories required by the sedentary modern man. You will read later about the health benefits of physical exercise, but for now, the extra food eaten by the labourer meant a higher actual quantity of foods consumed. Not only that, but our hard-working ancestor would eat a lower proportion of nutrient-weak foods such as the cakes and biscuits and white bread that we eat today – there were few refined carbohydrates around, less rushed eating, and less snacking. The cattle were the ones grazing, and doing so on nutrient rich grasses. This was the final advantage our ancestor held over us – his food was much richer in fats, proteins, minerals and vitamins. The accumulated effect of these factors would mean that the labourer was probably consuming at least 3 times as many minerals and vitamins as the modern office worker.

And enough fats to ensure that these nutrients were properly assimilated.
ww

In its subjugation of food quality for quantity, Big Food is also guilty of sub standard animal treatment. This is cruel to the animals, who frequently suffer mental illness. In addition, the animals incur physical problems as a result of ludicrously cramped living conditions. But more pertinently, such 'damaged' animals are more likely to yield poor quality milk, eggs and meat. This is a very well documented problem, and extensively covered elsewhere.

Instead, I want to finish this chapter with some light at the end of the dark tunnel we appear to be in. The book and film "Food Inc." [FI] discuss a breath of fresh air in the form of an American organic yogurt business called Stony Field Dairy. They risked much higher prices than their competition by using the highest-quality food sources, adherence to good environmental practices, a healthy work place, and 10% of profits given to worthy causes each year. In spite of strong warnings that this virtuous business approach was doomed to failure, they became highly successful, achieving consistent and healthy yearly growth, and good shareholder dividends. The bottom line was that the public were very happy to pay extra for extra quality. It also showed that the greed centric business 'norm' is not the only route to success.

Chapter Ten

Native diets

The large scale consumption of grains is a relatively recent event in the millions of years that humans have wandered the Earth. It would appear that around 40,000 years ago, humans started migrating from the hunter gatherer roaming lifestyle to a more settled one. It is likely that the group social benefits of community life that encampments provided, such as a more protective and nurturing environment for offspring, started outweighing the vulnerability of a fixed abode. It is indeed likely that the arrival of agriculture and domestication of animals followed this settling process, rather than catalysed it.

Certainly, larger groups gathered together were more likely to prosper, and their burgeoning numbers would look to the plentiful and more reliably obtained foods of cultivation. Agriculture is reckoned to have started around 12,000 years ago, some tens of thousands of years after tribes first started to settle. The exact figure is in dispute, however, and is of course likely to vary considerably across the globe anyway.

A probably-unforeseen downside of these settlements was the fast spread of illness, but by the same token, they had greater collective abilities to tend for the sick. Large communities also had greater synergy, and became more adaptive to change. Indeed, the reduced need to hunt saw a shift from brawn to brain, where social capabilities became much more important in the larger and richer community life that was evolving. It might be surprising to know that communication and social skills are very demanding on the brain.

As numbers grew, the erratic supply of hunted animal foods was supplemented more and more by plant food, and dairy products from grazing animals. Around 10,000 years ago, grains were adopted as an additional food source to feed increasing numbers of people. Such a source of food was previously mostly rejected because of the labour intensive nature of reaping – no combine-harvesters to ease the process at that time. And it is not enough to reap grains – they also have to be heated to break down the grain cell walls in order that the content be properly digestible.

Whilst 10,000 years is but a moment in the long history of humans, it is likely to have been enough to see a genetic adaption that allowed the grains to be assimilated well – enabling grain to be eaten in addition to animal products. More precisely, whole grains. And that means that the husk was included, even when ground to make breads (except that is, in China, where the husks have always traditionally been removed from rice). The modern process of refinement removes the husk, leaving white grains, depleted of minerals and vitamins and fibre, and much faster to digest than whole grains, which were in turn faster to digest than meat. And most humans (apart from maybe in eastern countries), have only had decades rather than centuries to adjust to such 'fast' food. Native diets, in general, were based on a mix of animal foods and mineral and vitamin rich whole grains.

Moving on to the beginning of the 19th century, it is important to note that cancer, the blight of the modern world, was a rarity. Approximately only 1 in 50 people in the western world got cancer. Whilst the number may have been higher than this as a result of weaker detection and diagnosis, cancer was relatively uncommon. [TT] By the beginning of the 20th century, however, the number had doubled to around 1 in 27. One hundred years later, it had soared to around 1 in 3. At the time of writing, it is closer to 1 in 2. For such a devastating disease, this is of course alarming. As you will see, it would appear that refined carbohydrates are the most guilty culprit for cancer growth, along with many other degenerative diseases.

In 1913, when medical man Albert Schweitzer started work in South Africa, there were no known incidences of death by cancer. This all changed when the native diet was partially displaced by a Western diet, replete with refined carbohydrates, and serves to illustrate the problem. But one anecdote does not make a good case for a causal relation. Fortunately, native diets came under the spotlight in the mid 20th century.

In the 1930's, an explorer named Stefansson spent no less than 10 years living with Eskimos, who at the time still adhered to a largely invariant native diet. Not that they had much choice of course – with virtually no food stuff arriving into the North Pole, they had to be self sufficient. Which meant a diet consisting almost exclusively of fish and sea mammals such as seals. As a rare visitor, and destined to stay years rather than days, Stefansson was obliged to eat like a native. At first, he struggled to eat the daily fare of fatty muscle and organ meats, but eventually adjusted. What surprised him was not so much that he was able to tolerate such a monotonous diet, and one that fundamentally lacked fruit and vegetables, but that he grew to thrive on it, both in the sense of taste and the ensuing elevation of physical health. He had suffered headaches for years and these gradually faded away.

Upon his return to the US, Stefansson returned to an American diet, but espoused the virtues of the Eskimo diet. So much so that he agreed to undertake a year long experiment with a colleague, Anderson, both eating 'only' 2 pounds of fatty meat a day for a full year whilst under the close scrutiny of physicians and dieticians. It was evident within a few weeks that these two men did indeed adhere to this diet, and were obviously none the worse for doing so. At the end of a year completely free from fruit and vegetables, the physicians could find no health issues with them.

At around the same time, an eminent dentist by the name of Weston Price was asking colleagues about research into healthy teeth and jaws. He found it not just a curiosity, but alarming that dental practices were based on an understanding of bad dental health rather than good. To his dismay, he discovered that there was a paucity of material on healthy teeth and jaws. Yet he was of course aware that many so-called 'primitive' tribes presented flawless, immaculate looking teeth. He was rightly alarmed that it had become standard practice to brutally drill into failing teeth, rather than look to cure or prevent the caries that caused them in the first place. As a man of action, he did not let the matter rest, and set off around the world in search of examples of good dental health, a journey that would take the better part of ten years.

His first port of call was with the people of the Loetschental valley in Switzerland in 1931. [ND] It was an opportune time to visit since a new motorway under construction at the time provided access to this community who had essentially been isolated for centuries. The 2,000 or so residents existed on a diet unchanged for generations. Cattle grazing on luscious green pastures (that were found to have very high vitamin and mineral contents) yielded very rich milk that was necessarily consumed in its raw state, along with butters and cheeses eaten with rye bread. The children who grew up on this simple fare (that was occasionally accompanied by meats) were big, strong, and radiantly healthy. For his own particular sphere of interest, Price noted universally wide jaws, with very little tooth crowding and very low levels of tooth decay. These wide jaws and nostrils also enhanced breathing.

Any suspicions that the high quality of health of these Swiss could be attributed more to genetics than nutrition were foiled by knowledge of those natives who left and subsequently returned to the valley. Such locals who departed and adopted a Western diet, laden with refined carbohydrates and with lower levels of minerals and vitamins, invariably suffered dental caries. Upon return, the degradation in health was arrested when the native diet was resumed.

As a result of this and his subsequent travels to many remote areas of the world, Price determined that good nutrition was not only key to good dental health, but that its influence reached much, much further than dental matters. From his observations, he determined that a poor diet, especially one high in refined carbohydrates, was the likely cause of narrow jaws, sinuses and nostrils in offspring. More controversially, Price was able to deduce an affect of refined foods on mental health. He noted that around 80% of mentally ill people had palatial deformities compared to around 20% of mentally healthy people. [ND] These deformities, especially the narrowing of the jaw, would appear to be a consequence of poor head development caused by a shortage of the right foods from the mother during pregnancy. There were samples in his travels of wide jawed parents with narrow-jawed offspring when a 'Western diet' was adopted. A drastic physiological change in just one generation. [ND]

The findings of Price were profound. In order to preserve and enhance them, the Weston A. Price Foundation was established. Their web site **www.westonaprice.org** is a rich store of health advice, untainted by big industry influence, and well worth exploring.

In the 1960's, the Tokelau people lived principally on just coconuts and fish, but were in robust health. Until the 1970's, that is, when the introduction of Western foods also saw an explosion in diseases. The Masai tribe in Africa principally eat meat, blood and milk, sometimes consuming over a pound of buttermilk, yet have no incidences of heart-disease or cancer. G. T. Wrench reported in 1938 on the Hunza peoples, big and strong, also living on a traditional diet. [WH] Note that their ripe health may have been at least partly down to the cultivation of soil that was lubricated with glacial mineral water.

And here we see the two key factors in good nutritional health – nutrient enrichment via good soil, and the avoidance of refinement that yields nutrient impairment. Good nutritional health is a much richer subject than these two factors of course, but they lay down a solid foundation for good health through the food you eat. Food derived from poor soils is low in nutrients. Refine it and you denude it further. So we often eat food that has been doubly stripped of nutritional value, and which is also too fast to assimilate for the good of the body.

The most worrying type of carbohydrate refining is that of sugar cane. The removal of the nutritional component of the cane (sold on as molasses) leaves familiar white sugar. Sugar is the extreme form of refinement, and is assimilated extremely fast, thereby destabilising homeostasis (the balance of the bodily systems). But the problem is aggravated by another factor. The metabolism of sucrose requires vitamins E and B1, and the body's supplies are cannibalised when sugar is consumed without them. Sugar consumed in isolation – such as in a sweetened drink – is hence a negative source of these vitamins. You may receive energy from the sugar, but you deplete your body of nutrients in the process.

Price (and others) concluded that degenerative diseases, including the aforementioned cancer, are mostly caused by nutritional deficiencies. It is logical, then, to turn attention in more detail to nutrition.

Chapter Eleven

Nutrition and digestion

You have seen even in my brief history of nutritional health advice that we have been regularly misinformed. It is time to cover some of the basics of nutrition, and dispel some of the untruths. Your health is highly correlated with what you eat, so a clearer understanding is paramount to optimal health.

The degree with which your diet affects you is easily underestimated. To illustrate quite how far reaching the effects of nutrition are on our health, it is worth touching on a new multidisciplinary science called Nutrigenomics, which is concerned with the interaction between food and genetics. It is a three fold matter. First, how food affects gene expression. Second, how food can affect the physical gene structure. And third, how genetics affects the way food is digested. Whilst this subject is mostly beyond the scope of this book, it is worth knowing that our genetic profile and genetic expression can affect how food is assimilated. Not only this, but that what we eat can affect us in a more sustained way than might be imagined because it can bring about genetic changes! By way of example, research on mice has shown that the diet of the mother during gestation can effect the epigenome of her offspring – the genetic inheritance of her offspring – resulting in mutations in some cases. For further, see :

http://learn.genetics.utah.edu/content/epigenetics/nutrition/.

A component of the third aspect of nutrigenomics, where our genetics affects how we digest and process food, is essentially our metabolism. As mentioned before, and as confirmed by research, [DD] many obese people are genetically predisposed to have low basal metabolic rates. Additionally, they have an impaired adipose fat tissue release mechanism, a condition named Lipophilia. As the aforementioned research on low-calorie diets has shown, obese people cannot raise their metabolism to compensate for overeating. And the fat they store is reluctantly released from their fat cells. This is largely linked with an adipose tissue enzyme called adipocate phospholipase A_2 (AdPLA). Research showed rodents with low levels remained lean even when on very high fat diets (Nature Magazine, 11th January 2009),

Only a slight metabolic imbalance is enough to create an ongoing weight gain, and as weight is gained, and the genetically unlucky person becomes obese, mobilising a larger body becomes a burden, thereby exacerbating their plight. A plight that is also aggravated further by the stigma associated with obesity. There appears to be strong evidence that many obese may actually be suffering a constant state of starvation in order to achieve a stable weight. This may sound absurd, but when adipose fat storage (lipogenesis) is genetically favoured over adipose fat release (lipolysis), then a tendency to gain weight is inevitable, even where the imbalance is tiny.

Those that believe that obesity can be remedied by strictly following a low-calorie diet miss this point entirely. In their defence, the low-calorie diet supporters cite the 1st law of thermodynamics as the scientific basis for advocating calorie reduction :

Energy in = Energy stored + Energy expended

This is, of course, not under debate, although it cannot strictly be applied to food and its digestion since energy from food that is not stored is not *all* expended as energy. Some is excreted via the skin, respiratory system, bladder and bowels. So food essentially takes three routes – storage within the body in adipose and other body cells, expenditure as work performed by and within the body, and the expulsion of the remainder.

But the biggest misunderstanding about the application of this law is to assume that the left hand side of the equation is the driving force.[DD] The arrival of food within your body is but a part of the of the fat storage and energy release processes. Lipogenesis and lipolysis are a constantly operating partnership. The driving force is not the arrival of food, but the propensity of the body to store the food as fat or utilise it as energy. And this – our metabolic nature – is wildly variant from person to person. The same food eaten by one person can be processed entirely differently by another.

Consider an analogy where money replaces food. A cautious person would likely save (store) a lot and spend (expend) a little, whereas a more reckless person would save little for a rainy day and spend heavily today. If these propensities were genetic, then the cautious person would get increased savings (fatten) given more money (food), whereas the reckless person would struggle to save more (they would stay thin) when given more money – simply spending (expending) the excess.

Lean people tend to burn off excess calories as heat and energy, via a rise in metabolic rate. Many obese people preferentially store food as fat (saving for a rainy day as it were).

The cells of the body create the energy demands that result in a rise in appetite. If these cells are not furnished the energy they need because much food is being stored as fat instead, then the appetite can remain unfulfilled. Hence the likelihood to gain weight, or to remain weak and hungry for much of the time if weight is kept stable. The fault is with the genetic predisposition more than with the habits or discipline of the obese person. The energy in (left had side of the equation) is not the driving force.

There is another factor that appears to blight the lives of the obese. In the non-obese, as adipose fat cells increase in size, they release Leptin, which curbs the appetite. This process is governed by the ob gene, a gene that appears to be missing in many obese people, meaning that they really cannot stop getting fat as they remain permanently hungry.

I mentioned earlier that dietary research with obese subjects concluded that a low-carbohydrate diet was not only effective at achieving weight loss, but that the subjects generally did not suffer the ill effects experienced on low-calorie diets. In terms of the body chemistry, most of the triglycerides in adipose fat cells are generated from dietary carbohydrates. A by-product of carbohydrate metabolism is glycerol phosphate, high levels of which promote fat storage as triglycerides, where the glycerol phosphate becomes the binder. The release of these triglycerides as energy in the form of free fatty acids (FFAs) is affected by the level of sugar in the blood. High blood sugar levels and high glycerol phosphate levels tend to block the FFA release. A reduction in carbohydrate intake, and hence a reduction in blood sugar level surges, can not only limit fat storage, but also enhance fat release as FFAs. A rebalancing of nutrients, favouring energy from fats over carbohydrates can paradoxically assist in weight loss.

A paradox of course because fat, and in particular saturated fat, has acquired a very bad name for over half a century now. Some indication of the importance of saturated fat, however, can be found in the high quantities found in the initial food we consumed as well fed babies – breast milk.

The first point to note about saturated fats is that they do not oxidise, and are thus very stable, unlike monounsaturated and polyunsaturated fats, which do oxidise and are less stable. It is, alas, the latter that the public are being steered towards. Saturated fats are required for cell wall structural stability. But there are also other properties of saturated fats that are conveniently forgotten. The consumption of saturated fats reduce stress hormone levels. Conjugated linoleic acid, lauric acid and capric acid, all found in saturated fats, have anti-cancer properties. Yet it is fat, and not refined carbohydrates, that is indicted as a cancer cause. As D. T. Cleave stated so eloquently :

"For a modern disease to be related to an old fashioned food is one of the most ludicrous things I ever heard in my life".

87

Malignant tumours are inaerobic – they are greedy for glucose – and consume up to 5 times the amount a normal cell would use. Replace some carbohydrates with fats in your diet and you start to starve cancerous cells because fats and proteins are aerobically processed.

Ironically, an often forgotten recommendation from both the Food and Agriculture Organisation (FAO) and the World Health Organisation (WHO) is that the recommended fat consumption dietary ratio of Polyunsaturated Fat Acid (PUFA) to Saturated Fatty Acid (FSA) is 0.6 : 1.0. Saturated fat intake should exceed polyunsaturated fat intake. But this is rarely the case when the vegetable oil industry coerces us to preferentially use their products. We are directed towards the wrong foods, and advisory bodies succumb to industry pressure to keep quiet about their own guidance that contradicts this direction.

Prime targets for scare mongering are eggs and meat, yet both actually contain more monounsaturated fat than saturated fat. Red meat contains around 50% monounsaturated fat and 45% saturated fat. The latter contains 15 percentage units of stearic acid, which is converted by the liver to monounsaturated fat in the form of oleic acid. Red meat is also high in creatine for muscle building.

Fats in general are also vital for the absorption of micronutrients such as fat soluble vitamins A, D, E and K. If you eat a salad containing the beneficial ingredients carotenoids and lycopene, they will not be assimilated properly without fat. Fat in the diet is also vital for sustaining healthy oil levels in the skin. I personally suffered with much dry skin in all the years that I cut off every last bit of fat from my meat. Within a few weeks of increased fat intake, my skin developed a lustrous, silky smooth feel.

Possibly as a result of their tendency to oxidise, research has linked polyunsaturated fats to cancer. [TT] However, in small quantities, they are actually vital to the body, for example to give cell walls their flexibility. And there is one type of polyunsaturated fat that has already been mentioned as very beneficial to our health – omega 3 – the best source of which apparently is sardines. Both omega 3 and omega 6 fatty acids are converted to ecosanoids, which are used in many cell reactions.

However, omega 3 and omega 6 essentially work in opposite directions, and the balance of their quantities in the diet is probably more important than their absolute values. The ratio of omega 6 to omega 3 was around 2:1 in Paleolithic times, and this is likely to be the ideal ratio for optimum health. However, the modern ration tends to err towards to 6:1, with deleterious effects.

As has already been mentioned already, a big target of the drug industry is cholesterol. The treatment of 'high cholesterol' is via a group of drugs called statins, which earn Big Pharma billions of dollars a year. It is so high a revenue earner that they of course push to lower the threshold at which it is prescribed. You are likely to be recommended a statin if your cholesterol level is too high, even if the blood test that revealed this was intended for another purpose. The claim is that high cholesterol levels correlate with heart disease, yet this is not born out by research results. [DD] (High triglyceride levels, resulting from high carbohydrate intake, *has* however been shown to correlate with heart-disease). [TT] Nor was a correlation found between cholesterol levels and cancer. [DD]

In Japan in 1980, methods for *raising* cholesterol levels was sought since the opposite situation of low cholesterol was causing too many strokes. Statins are pushing millions of unwary people in that direction, where they also incur many other ailments, such as memory loss, and muscular problems. Cholesterol is vital to the body, yet many of us are told to take statins, which interfere with the enzyme used in the synthesis of cholesterol in the liver. Statins lierally block a vital operation of the body. One of the more insidious side effects of statins is that they also lower levels of Co-Enzyme Q10 (CoQ10), which is vital for cellular Adenosine Triphosphate (ATP) energy generation. And ATP is a a vital energy for most cells of the body.

More recently, low cholesterol products and cholesterol lowering products have started appearing on the supermarket shelves. The aim of lowering your cholesterol by consuming less cholesterol is relatively pointless. The average person synthesises around 1,000 mg a day, some

3 times the amount normally consumed in the diet. The amount synthesised is modified anyway according to the amount in the diet.

The fundamental reality is that cholesterol is vital to the healthy functioning of the human body. Developing babies need copious amounts for eye and brain development. Human breast milk is high in cholesterol, in addition to the enzyme required for its digestion. Powdered baby milk is very low in cholesterol because of the tarnishing of the cholesterol name by industry, and is consequently damaging to the baby's growth. It is vital for cell membrane permeability and fluidity. Brain cells are crucially dependent on cholesterol, as is the immune system. Cholesterol is involved in the manufacture of hormones that help keep the skin hydrated. Serotonin re-uptake in the brain requires cholesterol – a shortage can lower serotonin effectiveness and possibly lead to depression. It is no small surprise that low cholesterol levels correlate with suicide and violence. [PP]

It might be prudent to see cholesterol as you would adrenaline. Would you be happy to take a tablet if your doctor measured your adrenaline levels and claimed they were too high? Maybe you could tell him that your adrenaline levels are high because you are excited about a new TV arriving that afternoon. Or that you are anxious about seeing the doctor in the first place. Adrenaline levels are always varying. Adrenaline, like cholesterol, is vital to the body. When we are under stress, cholesterol is released by the liver to deal with some of the consequences, such as free radicals. If your physician were to measure your cholesterol at such a time, and prescribe a statin he is failing in two senses. First, to mistake a temporary symptom as a long term one. Second, to fail to determine exactly *why* the level is high. Again, the adherence to the overly simplistic symptom-drug relationship is failing the patient here. Most cardiac arrest is caused by arrhythmia, in turn caused by stress, and not fat or cholesterol levels. The long running Framington study found that when cholesterol levels were lower in subjects, they were more likely to die younger.

Cholesterol requires a transport mechanism in order to travel through the watery bloodstream. The five types of transport are :

- High Density Lipoproteins (HDLs)
- Low Density Lipoproteins (LDLs)
- Very Low Density Lipoproteins (VLDLs)
- Intermediate density Lipoproteins (IDLs)
- Chylomicrons

HDLs are deemed the hero, sweeping up excess cholesterol, and returning it to the liver, and LDLs the villain, taking cholesterol to arteries, where it is claimed to build up on the walls, leading to atherosclerosis. LDL levels are generally not normally directly measured since specialised equipment is required to measure them accurately. Instead, they are calculated from HDL measurements. But this misses the key point. Robert Krauss pointed out in 1980 that LDLs come in 7 types, and that it was the smallest of these that correlated most with heart-disease. [DD] All LDLs are packaged in a single apo B protein. The correlation to heart disease is not with the amount of LDL cholesterol cargo, but with the high number of very small LDLs required to transport it. Too much apo B protein is the problem. Measuring total LDL, especially indirectly, is too crude a guide to cardiovascular vulnerability.

So the message that LDLs are bad, and HDLs are good is overly simple. Not all LDLs are bad. A diet high in carbohydrates increases the proportion of small LDLs, and hence increases the chance of heart disease. Additionally, high levels of carbohydrates also yields high VLDL levels, also correlated with heart disease.

And finally, to salt. 'The salt of the earth', 'He is worth his salt', as the sayings used to go, but now, sadly, salt is a food that has acquired a guilty label. Yet it is vital for health. In recent years, however, salt is coupled with fat as a baddie, and a lowering of consumption is strongly recommended. But no link has so far been found between salt intake and hypertension. [TT] Besides, an excess consumption of salt is excreted. When consumption is low, the kidneys retain salt. These regulatory mechanisms mean that we should not be overly concerned by the total amount of salt consumed. However, salt can be addictive, and whilst excessive intake will eventually be flushed from the body, until it is, it can raise blood pressure, so limit the amount at any one meal.

Nutrition is, of course, intimately linked with digestion, and it would be remiss of me to omit this matter. When I first read 'Gut Reaction' by Gudrun Jonsson, [GR] I was amazed to learn that we have, in effect, a second brain in our gut. It is called the enteric nervous system, and comprises around 100 million neurons. A tiny number in comparison to the brain in our heads, but nevertheless, an independent intelligence that manages the gut in the tissues lining the oesophagus, stomach, small intestine and colon. It controls the rate of digestion, digestive secretions, and muscular contractions along the gut.

The vagus nerve connects the two brains together, and we are in greatest health when the two operate in concert. Note that the vagus nerve is implicated in emotional health, and it is therefore no surprise that our 'gut feelings' have some neurological basis. But the presence of an additional brain in the gut has much more profound repercussions. When we pop a pill that is 'targeted' at our brain, it is a truism, of course that the pill does not know the target. It will necessarily indiscriminately affect both the brain in our head and the one in our guts, with potentially dire consequences such as diarrhoea and constipation. These are deemed occasional side-effects of many drugs, but this hides the reality that a drug is no silver bullet, homing in on just the desired target area. It will always affect the whole body indiscriminately. Such a side effect is in fat one of the *actual* effects of a drug.

Digestion starts in the mouth, where all too many of us fail to chew food properly. The commonly held view is that we should chew in order to break down the food into small pieces for better digestion. This is partly true, but there are two other key benefits gained from slowly chewing food. (And yes, I agree that many foods these days are so soft that it is almost impossible to chew for long). First, that sustained chewing allows the saliva enzymes to work on the food. Secondly that the release of these enzymes triggers the stomach into preparing itself for an onslaught of food. If the food arrives too rapidly, the stomach is ill prepared, and a stomach ache can ensue.

Another extremely common modern habit concerning food is that we often eat too fast, and often whilst at our desks at work. Just as a slow, repeated chewing of food is crucial to good digestion, a relaxed attitude is vital. If you are engrossed in work, then blood is diverted away from the stomach, again compromising its operation. It appears that eating food with the right attitude aids digestion. [AI]

Pints of acids in the stomach start to break down digested food, which then travels to the small intestine where it is broken down further and absorbed through the intestinal walls. Note that in essence, the digestive tract is external to the body, much like the hole in a doughnut. Absorption is a carefully controlled process – the body allows only what it deems safe through the intestinal walls.

The pancreas is the organ of digestion. It adds alkali to neutralise the broken down food mix, along with insulin to marshal sugar in the blood to muscle or fat cells. It also secretes a number of enzymes – Proteases to break down protein, Amylases to break down starch, and Lipases to break down fat. The pancreas works in concert with the gall bladder, which releases bile to emulsify fat before the pancreatic lipase enzymes work to split the fat into sizes small enough to enter the bloodstream.

Along the way, the stomach absorbs sugar, alcohol, and water soluble vitamins. The small intestine absorbs the remaining food nutrients, leaving the large intestine to recover water from the mix. It is crucial here to note that carbohydrates are rapidly processed by the stomach. Note that carbohydrates are all essentially sugars – complex carbohydrates are simply long chains of sugar molecules – whose break-down yields glucose. Note also that table sugar is sucrose – a combination of glucose and fructose (fruit sugar). Proteins and fats stay longer in the stomach, and are used to indicate when you are getting full. [S1] Fat is the key indicator of satiety. Since carbohydrates are processed rapidly by the stomach, an excess can be eaten without feeling full.

I mentioned earlier that Vitamins A, D, E and K require fat for assimilation. Mineral absorption requires both fat and these Vitamins for assimilation. Vitamin A is required for protein assimilation.

There is another indictment on these poor carbohydrates. MIT researchers Dr Judith Wurtman and Dr Richard Wurtman found that serotonin was released during carbohydrate digestion. [DI] There is a subsequent serotonin drop to accompany the more well know fall in blood sugar as insulin released by the pancreas moves it to body cells. The combination of the two creates uncomfortable feelings that are readily rectified by the consumption of more carbohydrates. So carbohydrates are in effect an addictive food. This effect is similar to that caused by alcohol and tobacco, both established addictive substances of course. Conversely, fat as fuel results in stable serotonin and blood sugar levels. The post lunch lethargy of a carbohydrate rich meal is generally not observed in a fat-rich meal.

Not only is glucose the fuel that some cancers feed on, but insulin is also required for tumour growth. US Geneticist Howard Martin Temin won the Nobel prize in 1975 for discovering this. [DD] Malignant breast cancer cells have more Insulin Growth Factor (IGF) receptors, so are particularly active in the presence of high insulin levels. [DD] Even minor matters such as acne are affected by raised insulin levels. During puberty, androgen levels are raised – insulin raises them further, flooding skin pores, with the resultant visual impairments.

In an attempt to reduce sugar consumption, many overweight people use artificial sweeteners. The December 2009 edition of the British magazine New Scientist gave some revealing insights into the effect of sweeteners. Psychologist Guido Frank at the University of Colorado in Denver used functional Magnetic Resonance Imaging (fMRI) to observe the brain of subjects when eating either sucrose or the sweetener Sucralose. The sucrose activated the reward centre, in effect increasing satiety. The sucralose had a much lower effect. Further studies indicated that the brain is able to detect the lack of calories in the sweetener. Yet the sweetener creates a strong sweet taste. The mind is expecting calories but gets none, so appears to crave the missing calories.

But sweeteners are not just passive chemicals. It is well established that the sweetener Aspartame essentially failed in drug testing, causing brain damage to rats. But the results were suppressed and it was approved (search for 'aspartame' on www.westonprice.org). Criminally, for such a dangerous chemical, its approval has been elevated to a status so trusted that it is often excluded in the US from the list of ingredients of foods where it is used as an additive. Additionally, aspartame also contains the amino acid Phnelalanine which is known to lower serotonin levels, and hence create a food craving.

As mentioned much earlier, fruits and vegetable are lumped together in the generic advice for a daily consumption of 5 or more portions. But the principle sugar in fruits is fructose. Part of the reason that table sugar has a lower glycemic index than glucose is because of the fructose it contains. (The glycemic index is a guide to the speed of absorption of foods. The lower the number, the slower the food is to digest, and the less harmful, in general, it is to the stability of our metabolism). Fructose is not processed by the stomach – it is transported to the liver for processing, so it does not affect blood sugar directly. It does not require pancreatic insulin for assimilation. The liver converts it into triglycerides, an excess of which is deleterious to health.

Additionally, fructose is responsible for elevating blood pressure. [DD] Fructose also appears to be responsible for the formation of advanced glycation end products (AGE), and the oxidisation of LDL cholesterol, both of which are harmful to health. [DD] It is also an indicator for insulin resistance, which can lead to diabetes. In the light of such knowledge, fruit is not quite the super healthy food that it is made out to be. And it certainly does not deserve to have the same standing as vegetables.

The processing of carbohydrates results in a surge in blood sugar (glucose) levels. This triggers the beta cells in the islets of Langerhans in the pancreas to release insulin, an anabolic hormone, whose function is to regulate energy and glucose metabolism in the body. Insulin transports the glucose to the liver, muscles and fat cells, whose insulin receptors allow the glucose to be absorbed. The presence of insulin also suppresses the release of fat from adipose tissue.

The lower levels of insulin is key to the efficacy of a low-carbohydrate diet. When carbohydrate levels are reduced, not only is less glucose converted to triglycerides and stored in fat cells, but the body shifts to a use of FFAs (Free Fatty Acids), more readily released from adipose tissue in the absence of insulin. It is in a sense a paradox that the dietary replacement of carbohydrates with fat can result in an increase in lipolysis. Eating fat can cause the release of fat from fat cells. Just ponder that for one moment. Dietary carbohydrates cause body fat to be laid down, dietary fat causes body fat to be released. Additionally, a prominence of fat in the diet results in a very steady blood sugar level, and a greater feeling of satiety. Eat a high-fat, low-carbohydrate meal slowly, and you will feel fuller for much longer than on a low-fat, high-carbohydrate meal of the same calorific value.

When large quantities of carbohydrates are consumed often enough, the body cells are under a sustained bombardment of high insulin levels. Eventually, the insulin receptors on these cells can lose their sensitivity. They become insulin resistant. As a consequence, they take up less glucose, so more insulin is released as the body strives to clear the blood stream of excess glucose. This insulin resistance is called type 2 diabetes. If high carbohydrate levels are sustained, the resistance increases, and insulin levels increase, placing a growing load on the pancreas. Eventually, the beta cells can fail, and the effects of diabetes starts to manifest in physical symptoms. The ever high insulin levels make retrieval of fat from adipose tissue ever harder, leading to obesity. It is much more likely that obesity is a consequence rather than a cause of diabetes. Type 2 diabetes is referred to as late onset diabetes, as it normally takes effect later in life.

Type 1 diabetes, a much more serious condition, generally starts suddenly in early life, and is referred to as early onset diabetes. It appears to be an immune system failure, where the beta cells are attacked by the body. Their depleted numbers mean that less and less insulin can be produced by the pancreas, resulting in dangerously high blood sugar levels. Conventionally, insulin is injected by type 1 sufferers to make up for the shortfall. A type 1 diabetic can also get type 2 diabetes if high levels of carbohydrates are consumed.

There is a theory that the immune system starts attacking the beta cells as a direct response to sustained high insulin levels. [ON] And that a low-carbohydrate, adequate-protein, very-high-fat diet – so called Optimum Nutrition – can actually cure type 1 diabetes. [ON] Certainly, for both forms of diabetes, a low-carbohydrate diet appears to be essential.

Note that exercise enhances beta cell production. [PA] It also improves insulin sensitivity by adding new insulin receptors to body cells. [SP] I personally suffer with hypoglycaemia, or low blood sugar. (The high blood sugar level of type 1 diabetes is termed hyperglycaemia). Following the blood-sugar rise resulting from an intake of carbohydrates, and the subsequent drop courtesy of insulin, the hypoglycaemic subsequently either suffers too rapid or too deep a blood-sugar drop (or a see-saw effect in some cases).

Alas, Hypoglycaemia is rarely ever diagnosed, even though I believe that it is likely to be a precursor to type 2 diabetes. It is often seen as an attitude problem rather than a real health issue. But the symptoms are significant and distressing, including :

- Confused thinking
- Irritability
- Intense craving for food
- Tremors/weakness/fainting
- Mood swings
- Fatigue
- Low self esteem from mood swings and irritability
- Drowsiness
- Headaches
- Anxiety etc

Note also that high carbohydrate levels means that cells preferentially choose glucose over Vitamin C, thereby creating a Vitamin C cellular shortage. Excessive carbohydrates are also implicated in syndrome X, a condition that can be a trigger for many ailments. This is a subject that is too involved for this book, but worth exploring on the Weston Price web site (www.westonaprice.org).

Chapter Twelve
Low carbohydrate diets

I will focus here on low-carbohydrate diets for the same reason that Gary Taubes did so in his brilliant book "The Diet Delusion" [DD] (better known as "Good Calories, Bad Calories" in the US). It is not just a key mechanism for reducing weight in the obese, and for countering the effects of diabetes, and for diminishing the effects of epilepsy, [KD] but a fundamental route to general good health for many (but not all) people. Not only can a diet low in fat result in such problems as eczema, gallstones, osteoporosis, and kidney damage, but the necessary high levels of carbohydrates used as the energy source in such a diet can create a plethora of conditions. Sustained high levels of carbohydrates, especially refined carbohydrates, sugars and fructose, can result in a swathe of degenerative diseases. [TT]

I feel strongly that the copious amount of confectionary I ate as a child was at least in part the cause for the appearance of osteoarthritis in both knee caps in my early 30's, my decades of hypoglycaemia and a large amount of tooth decay. In April 2009, after reading books on hypoglycaemia [HP] and diabetes [DI] I started to believe that I could gain better health by lowering the amount of carbohydrates I was currently eating, and favouring fats as the energy source. I must stress here that whilst this did indeed prove to be of great benefit to myself, a low-carbohydrate diet will not suit everyone. I cannot, and must not give a 'one-diet-suits-all' message. Explore for yourself what suits you and your metabolism.

Note that protein can be used as an energy source, but it is an inefficient one.

Dr Bernstein, an Engineer diagnosed with type 1 diabetes in 1946 aged 12 suffered a series of problems for 20 years on the then recommended high-carbohydrate diet. Frustrated at this decline in health, he used his engineering mindset and a very early blood sugar level device to micro-manage his insulin and food intake in order to attain a stable blood sugar level. This resulted in much lower insulin levels and a restoration of normal health. At the last count, he was maintaining his blood sugar at stable levels, living a healthy life into his 70's, exercising vigorously daily, and out living the majority of type 1 diabetics. [DI]

Reading the excellent book "Trick and Treat" by Barry Groves finally convinced me of the legitimacy of such a diet. Groves, a chemist, had adopted such a diet for decades, but was constantly ridiculed by colleagues, who were alarmed at the amount of fat he was consuming at each meal. That he was fit and healthy and perpetually slim, yet never went hungry was not enough to persuade them of the appropriateness and effectiveness of this diet. The fat-is-bad dogma has been so persuasive and pervasive for so many years now that it blinded them to the evidence of their own eyes.

Incensed by this ignorant stance, Groves eventually managed to work full time exploring the science behind this diet. His book is the result of no less than 26 years of full time, independent research. There is a great weight of evidence supporting the health benefits of a low-carbohydrate diet that he presents intelligently in his book. And if you are wondering about the title of his book, it refers to how we are tricked into eating refined carbohydrates and then treated for the ailments that result, a neat industry technique.

After starting to eating a low-carbohydrate, high-fat diet, the overall benefits were so profound that I have neither seen it as a 'diet', nor ever wanted to revert to my old eating habits. For someone who was plainly addicted to carbohydrates, who cut even the smallest amount of fat from meat, and refused to add gravy to meals, this was a radical change, and in hindsight, I suspect a gradual initial transition would have been wiser.

After a few days, my appetite all but disappeared, and the prospects of a full cooked English breakfast upon rising each morning created a sense of nausea. But I persisted of course, and now such a meal feels entirely natural.

By way of comparison, a typical hypoglycaemia driven daily regimen can be seen to be drastically different from this new way of eating, even though I had been eating relatively low levels of refined carbohydrates.

A typical day before diet change

08:00 Big bowl of porridge with milk and no added sugar

09:30 Food craving would see me eating a raw carrot

10:30 Food craving would see me eat a small peanut butter sandwich

11:30 And now an apple to tide me over until lunch

12:30 Fatless meat, rice and vegetables + chocolate

14:00 Food craving - ate half a banana

15:00 The other half of a banana

16:00 Maybe a few peanuts an a rice cracker

17:30 Fish, sweet potatoes, vegetables

19:30 Some peanuts, and maybe a couple of biscuits

21:30 Small bowl of porridge with milk for supper

A typical day on the new diet

08:00 Two poached free range eggs, one or two slices of bacon cooked in lard, a small piece of rye bread and a few peas cooked in butter

14:00 Meat with fat and added fats (such as butter, cream, goose fat) a small portion of sweet potatoes, and some spinach. A square of 80% cocoa chocolate and a little raw milk cheese as a pudding

20:00 Fish with coconut oil and olive oil, more sweet potatoes, and peppers, followed by a little more chocolate and cheese.

What is most evident is the difference in the number of hours between food intakes – the change of diet giving my stomach and digestive tract some rest. I am now generally simply not hungry between meals. It is of course no surprise when you see that my original breakfast, and a number of my snacks were very high in carbohydrates. I was also then consuming a larger volume of food, and quite probably more calories. The new diet has had the net effect of reducing my stomach size, and bodily fat levels. I certainly lost weight on a regular basis for the first 6 months or so. For someone driven by hypoglycaemic food cravings, eating every hour or 2 throughout the day, the ability to go for up to 7 hours without feeling the discomfort of gnawing hunger was delightful beyond words, and justification alone for continuing the diet. A life driven by frequent, intensely urgent bouts of eating is stressful. To be able to prepare a meal without that urgency to eat was ,and still is, a revelation. The rush to eat in order to relieve symptoms of irritability and light-headedness, cramming food into my mouth, was replaced by the pleasure of preparing a meal and then eating it at a slow pace. Unless you have experienced the discomfort of low-blood-sugar hunger, then it is difficult to convey how much a relief it was to put it behind me.

Looking back on my low-fat, high-carbohydrate lifestyle, there is one matter that frustrates me in hindsight. You see, I did occasionally eat a cooked breakfast instead of cereal, especially when on holiday. It sustained me for many hours, yet it never occurred to me that such a meal might be the best way to start every day. Likewise, a thick cheesy pizza at lunch would often leave me full until early evening, when I would have a light tea in the form of a banana sandwich, only to find myself hungrier within an hour than before I ate it. The fast sugars in such a sandwich, even with whole grain bread is a bad idea for a hypoglycaemic!

More subtle on the new diet was the stabilising not just of appetite but of mood. A fluctuating blood sugar level manifests in mood swings of one degree or other, even with my original regular eating pattern. Now, I am able to concentrate effortlessly for hours at a stretch. I have written some of this book for over 5 hours without a break and suffered no tiredness afterwards. My level of mental acuity has also increased. As someone who has additionally suffered tension headaches (since the mid 1990's), along with foggy thinking and tiredness, to see an improvement in all three of these was as welcome as much as it was unexpected.

Conversely, at the other extreme, the consumption of sugars fuels hyperactivity and lowers the ability to concentrate. A high-carbohydrate lunch can make you feel sleepy afterwards. I no longer suffer in this way. My energy levels have been raised in spite of (the initial few months of) weight loss. It bears no comparison with the persistent weakness and food-craving on low-calorie diets I experienced in the past.

In the early few days of the new diet, there were periods of light headedness that were probably a consequence of the rapidity of dietary change. There was also a hardening of faeces, and the consequential increase in bowel movement difficulties. These subsequently settled down, although I use a magnesium supplement to alleviate bowel movement difficulties if and when they reemerge. Much more important is that intestinal flora and yeasts were no longer so readily fuelled by carbohydrates, and bowel movements were no longer accompanied by noxious smells as a consequence. On most days, there is no obvious odour at all from bowel movements, nor any anal residue requiring cleansing. The change was like a breath of fresh air in more than the obvious sense. A toilet roll now lasted around 3 weeks, some-what longer than previously.

Whilst this is a taboo subject, it is necessarily a meaningful one for many people with anal irritations. I had suffered from this embarrassing and frustrating problem, colloquially termed 'the ring of fire', for many years. With the dietary change, it disappeared within a few days, presumably as a direct consequence of firmer stools leaving no residue. Because this is a subject that few feel able to talk about, those who suffer often do so in silence. At least this should help some of them.

Whilst I have always been naturally fairly slim, I was a little bit heavier at the start of this diet than I wanted to be. As you can see in figure 4 overleaf, my weight has varied over the years, as I have successfully dieted to attain a weight suitable for the sports I play, only for my it to gradually creep up over the months and years.

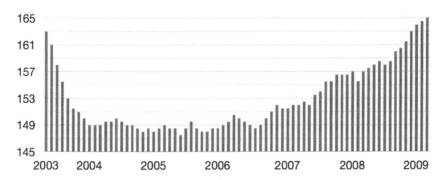

Figure 4 : Long term monthly average weight in pounds

Figure 5 below shows the first 6 months on the new diet. Remember that when adopting this diet, I was mostly eating when hungry, and not overtly looking to lose weight – I was not actively trying to lose anything more than a few pounds.

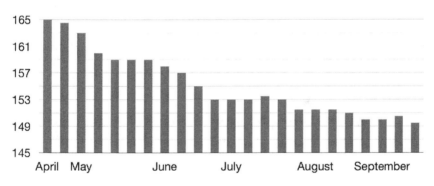

Figure 5 : Average weekly weight in pounds on low-carb diet

The fat-is-bad dogma is so ingrained, and the discrediting of the 'Atkins diet' with which it is inextricably linked is so strong, that many who might now seek to adopt this diet will not only be contending with concern from friends and family, but also from themselves! Even though I am often a determined man, and happy to break from convention, it took many months to feel that it was indeed safe and healthy to eat a high-fat diet, since I too was heavily influenced by the dogma.

Additionally, your physician is unlikely to endorse this diet, regardless of any obvious benefits it might bring. When I told my doctor that it had resolved health issues for myself, "That's good" was the only response I received. There was no enquiry.

How low should a low-carbohydrate diet go? Essentially, to the level where you reach and retain your ideal weight. But be wary that dropping below a certain level triggers a process called ketosis (not to be confused with diabetic ketoacidosis, a dangerous condition). The threshold varies from person to person, but is around 80 calories of pure carbohydrates a day for most people (note that 80 grams of potatoes, for example, contains fibre and water in addition to starch).

When glucose levels fall below a certain level, the body switches to using Free Fatty Acids (FFAs) as fuel. These are obtained from fat in the diet and from adipose fat cells, the latter readily released in the absence of insulin. With a low-carbohydrate diet, the pancreas switches from insulin to glucagon production, which triggers the liver to release glycogen stores and adipose cells to release FFAs. All but the brain can use FFAs as energy sources in the absence of glucose. When the liver breaks down FFAs, it creates ketone bodies as a by product. When these accumulate to high enough levels in the blood stream, the body is deemed to have entered ketosis. [KD]

The brain is entirely happy to switch from glucose to ketone bodies as an energy source. Up to 75% of its needs can be furnished from ketone bodies. De novo glucogenesis (new birth glucose) is a process that can furnish glucose from dietary protein when in ketosis to fuel the remaining 25% energy needs of the brain. Note that a ketogenic diet, where carbohydrate levels are low enough to switch the body into ketosis, is often slated as one prone to muscle wasting, but there are many who claim that it is a muscle protective diet, more so than low-calorie diets for example. [KD]

To optimise fat metabolism, especially if a life with a low-fat diet has preceded an adoption of the low-carbohydrate diet, it is advisable to take supplements. Chromium, Acetyl L-Carnitine and CoQ10 are recommended to assist the transition as they optimise fat metabolism.

The promotion of the low-carbohydrate diet by Atkins ushered in a stream of competing variations, cashing in on the obvious effectiveness of the diet. In order to differentiate themselves from Atkins, various aspects of human physiology were explored, along with varying proportions of fats, proteins and carbohydrates.

One key additional facet many books played upon was how human diversity affected dietary needs – the low-carbohydrate approach was seen as applicable only to certain types. Because the combinations of fat, protein and carbohydrates have such a bearing on our health, it is worth exploring a few of these alternatives. I leave detailed exploration to the referenced books.

In the "The Body Code", Jay Cooper [BC] latched onto soma typing, and glandular typing as a means of tuning the diet. The soma types are classifications of three basic body types. Ectomorphs are thin by nature, struggling to gain muscle mass. They essentially have a fast metabolism. I fall into this category. Endomorphs are like the polar opposite of Ectomorphs, having large frames, large muscle mass, readily gain fat, and have a slow metabolism. Mesomorphs lie inbetween, having athletic physiques, with powerful musculature, and low amounts of body fat. Cooper believes quite sensibly that we should eat according to our body type. Additionally, she believes that the relative strengths of our adrenal, gonad, thyroid and pituitary glands also has a strong bearing on how food affects us. For good measure, she also throws in Indian Ayurveda energy typing, and this is where it can get complex and fuzzy.

Cooper looks back to our ancestors to explain these soma, glandular and Ayurvedic origins. Whilst there is merit in accounting for these when determining diet, she synthesises from them four combinational human types – warrior, nurturer, communicator and visionary – and goes on to give low-carbohydrate diets tuned to each without explaining quite how she got to these neat four types in the first place. Nor does she explain the rationale behind her very detailed diets, making it hard to buy into her ideas.

The point here is that because advisory bodies are still stuck in the fat-is-bad groove, it is essentially left up to individual nutritionists and writers to give guidance to the public. With the lack of a guiding force, or regulatory mechanism, a lot of well intended, but sometimes misguided books like Cooper's eventually dilute and damage the potential genuine value of a low-carbohydrate diet.

"The Metabolic typing diet" by Wolcott and Fahey [MT] is a better disciplined book, exploring metabolic types and the balance between the sympathetic (fight and flight) and parasympathetic (rest and heal) nervous systems. Their belief is that eating in accordance with your body type, and with a respect of the balance of these complimentary nervous systems brings optimum health. They include a low-carbohydrate diet as the perfect route for certain types, but strongly believe that a high-carbohydrate diet is equally appropriate for other types.

That book provides both an interesting read and a timely caveat to the low-carbohydrate approach I have been focusing on. Just as peanuts are a perfect (albeit addictive) snack for some, for others, even a single nut can literally be fatal. The simple concept of one diet fitting all is ultimately as flawed as the universal nutritional advice that governments proffer to their public. Our constitutions and lifestyles vary so enormously that it would be incredible indeed if one size ever did fit all. The point is, however, that a low-carbohydrate diet has been shown by millions to be effective for a large percentage of the population. That it might not work for you does not negate its value for many.

According to D'Adamo and Whitney in "Eat right 4 your type", another physiological aspect is crucial to health. They believe, much as the Japanese do, that your blood type has a large bearing on both your health, and on how different foods affect you. Again, however, they appear to extrapolate on a whim from the four basic blood types to a set of diets highly tuned to each. It may well be that there are indeed interactions between certain foods and the constitutional variations that relate to the A, B, O and AB blood types. But they destroy their credibility with blatant inconsistency – for example, pork is decreed unsuitable for each of the blood types, but with no explanation supplied.

The glycemic index was a potentially pragmatic concept introduced by nutritional advisors to help people avoid the worst effects of eating carbohydrates. It allows them to know and thereby avoid foods which are assimilated most quickly by the body, and hence yield the most rapid rise in blood sugar levels. Rob Thompson used the glycemic index as the focus for his book "Glycemic load diet." [GL] But this approach is too narrow to be the only guidance for food intake. You may achieve slow assimilation of food, but without the right balance of nutrients, you will not attain optimum health.

In a series of books, Diana Schwarzbein promoted a variation of the low-carbohydrate diet followed in conjunction with a set of lifestyle guides. [S1, S2] Her more holistic approach makes more sense, and in essence follows the remit of the book you are reading – that good health is a balance of many factors. The low-carbohydrate variation she recommends seeks to get a more even balance between carbohydrates, fats and proteins. A lowish-carbohydrate diet. The lifestyle aspects of her books intelligently explores the balance of the sympathetic and parasympathetic nervous systems. Modern life is mostly spent in a driven state, engaging the (misleadingly named) sympathetic nervous system, in essence putting the restorative parasympathetic nervous system on hold. A key focus in her books is the balancing of hormone systems, since an imbalance is deemed to be key to accelerated body cell aging.

Eades and Groves took a different approach again in "The Protein Power Lifeplan." [PP] Their belief was that a low-carbohydrate diet high in protein was key to optimum health. Except that the book focuses almost exclusively on just the low-carbohydrate diet itself, and fails to supply a convincing argument for a high level of dietary protein. They do, however, revisit the impact of metabolism on dietary needs.

Working in the opposite direction, promoting just adequate levels of protein in a very high fat version of the low-carbohydrate diet is the Polish physician Dr Jan Kwaśniewski. [ON] Whilst he claims that his 'Optimum Nutrition' (ON) methodology is scientifically based, it was essentially developed empirically. As I have earlier stressed, the empirical approach has advantages over the scientific, not least in this case because Kwaśniewski spent no less than 30 years evolving his ideas, working on the many obese patients who visited his practice.

Testimony to his very high fat diet are the 2 million followers of it in Poland, where there are a few dozen doctors who recommend the diet to patients. An obvious feature of many ON practitioners is their slim appearance. Irena Kozlowicz had been suffering badly with knee problems aged 71. Seven years later on the diet she could bound up stairs like a 50 year old, her knee problems a thing of the past. Even the US city of Chicago has taken ON to its hearts, and has a restaurant for followers. Chicago physician Mark Sobor sees no problem with the diet – those patients of his on the diet are all slim, healthy and energetic. Another Chicago Physician, Christopher Kubik spent four years on the diet, moving from overweight and unhealthy to slim and healthy.

The scale of success of the ON diet cannot be denied – there are even two regular publications on the diet in newsagents in Poland. But Kwaśniewski appears to be an over-confident man, so much that he appears to be oblivious to certain details, not least the simple fact that no one diet can be universally suitable. His book claims a scientific approach, but fails to mention exactly what this science amounts to, nor how he derived his very precise 'optimum' combination of proteins, carbohydrates and fats. He would have been advised to admit that his combination was tuned empirically over the decades to be most universally efficacious with his patients. Even the combination in question is presented confusingly as :

$$Protein : Fat : Carbohydrate = 1 : 2.5\text{-}3.5 : 0.5$$

Much simpler and more accessible to round to whole numbers, and express as follows :

$$Protein : Fat : Carbohydrate = 2:5:1 \text{ up to } 2:7:1$$

He also fails to drive home the importance of measurement, and that all fat, protein and carbohydrates are found in most foods in varying combinations. Adhering to such a precise combination of food types becomes a logistical problem. At least, that is, until your body gets a feel of what makes an optimally balanced meal. For example, a beef steak has a P:F:C ratio of about 2:3:0. I would have assumed that protein would have been the dominant component.

Kwaśniewski claims to have cured type 1 diabetes via this diet to the point where insulin injections are no longer required. He also claims, (for which he presumably has detailed corroborating records), that the condition of low Lipase levels in obese patients is rectified given long enough on the diet. He claims that one lady who was bound to a wheelchair by multiple sclerosis was totally cured of her condition, and was eventually able to walk freely. An even more suspect claim is that he knows of no long time adopter of the diet who has become ill with cancer. It may well be that the low-carbohydrate levels starve cancers of life, but it seems unlikely that there is not one incidence of cancer in decades of administering the diet. Apparently Lech Walesa, the president of Poland lost 44 lbs of weight on the diet, curing himself of diabetes along the way.[ON]

Dr Przemyslaw Pala analysed the health of 6,000 ON practitioners over a period of 5 years, and found no negative health signs that could be attributable to the diet. He did find many ailments were resolved by the diet, including type 1 diabetes. In 2008, The Nutrition Research Journal number 28 reported on research on the diet. The paper was titled "Long-term consumption of a carbohydrate-restricted diet does not induce deleterious metabolic effects". The results are self evident, although the title obscures the fact that the subjects in the research were long term ON practitioners. A low-carbohydrate, *high-fat* diet.

If you find yourself in Poland, and see someone drinking a cup of double cream, do not be alarmed – it appears that it is actually beneficial for their health. Except, that is, that they are very strongly advised to drink it slowly!

Even if you do not adopt a consistent low-carbohydrate diet, you will see benefits from avoiding meals and snacks that are mostly carbohydrate in content, especially refined carbohydrates. There is an old proverb that says we should eat breakfast like a King, lunch like a Prince and dinner like a Pauper. The key point being to feed for the day ahead, not to load the belly with food overnight. And if breakfast is the most important meal, then my first recommendation would be that you replace a cereal and/or toast breakfast with at least a couple of free range eggs. You would then be giving your body a well balanced, long lasting start to the day. Maybe scrambled eggs on toast would be an ideal start for the day. If you cannot live without your toast, do not hold back on the butter – this will temper the fast assimilation of carbohydrates in the toast. And finally, do not hold back on fatty sauces and the fat on meat at lunch and dinner. It will keep you fuller for longer. And a greater dominance of fat in your diet may have its paradoxical effect of weight loss.

Chapter Thirteen

The benefits of exercise

It is time to move on from lengthy discussions of fuel for the body to the matter of how that fuel is used. Most obvious is physical exercise, a subject that has been under close scrutiny in recent years as we tend towards more and more sedentary lives. The pull of electronic devices is compelling, the TV now supplemented by games consoles and the Internet. How much easier to play tennis on your PC than it is to get changed, travel to the tennis courts, huff and puff your way round, shower and travel home. Yet the benefits of exercise generally compensate for the effort required.

Research has not only shown the obvious, that exercise is good for you, but that the benefit is generally proportional to the amount you do.[SP] As long as you can avoid injury and excessive stress on the body, then the more ongoing exercise the better. Note that the state of exercising is itself actually one of actual bodily stress, but generally a positive form of stress that ultimately strengthens more than it damages. The best exercises are those with a social context, which of course explains part of the popularity of sports. The very best exercises involve the mind, social bonding and mental agility. Activities such as Tai Chi, involving complex interactions with other people have been shown to stave off dementia.[BR]

The first health benefit of exercise relates to the general principle of human physiology – 'use it or lose it'. As you exercise, you direct the body to strengthen itself – to be able to cope with the demands of the exercise. Exercises like soccer, swimming and running tend to increase muscle bulk and strength, depending on your somatic type. Load bearing exercises strengthen both muscle and the bones, even in old age, providing greater all round structural strength and resilience. Note that muscle building does not actually occur during the exercise, but in the subsequent 24 hours, when the muscle is broken down and rebuilt a little stronger in response to the workout it has undergone.

The excellent book "Spark : the effect of exercise on the brain" [SP] shows that there is another very subtle effect of exercise :

"On a mechanical level, exercise relaxes the resting tension in muscle spindles, which breaks the stress-feedback loop to the brain. If the body isn't [physically] stressed, the brain figures maybe it can relax too [to stop mental stress]." (My brackets)

Research at Duke University in 2000 demonstrated that exercise was even superior to the anti-depression drug Sertralin (Zoloft) in alleviating depression. [SP] Even allowing for the loss of credibility that I have previously given to anti-depressant drugs, this still shows a valuable benefit for depressed people.

Pupils at Naperville Central High School in the US were the subject of an experiment that explored the practical consequences of a morning physical exercise regime. [SP] All children were obliged to run a mile before their first lesson. Surprisingly, this obligation was well received because the approach they adopted was an empathic, intelligent one. They had managed to buy a batch of heart-rate monitors that the children could wear during their run. Each child was to be rated according to the heart-rate elevation recorded by these devices, and thereby be rewarded for personal, individual effort.

Early on, they were able to make a surprising observation as a consequence of this approach. One child in particular was seen to be almost at a crawl when completing her mile. Their initial judgement was that she was simply not applying herself. Yet the heart rate monitor told an entirely different story. The run had tired her so much that even the slow pace at the end was pushing her heart-rate above 90% of maximum.

Each child was asked to run at 80% to 90% of maximum safe heart-rate, and rewarded according to their adherence to this, in conjunction with their running time. This had the profound effect of levelling the playing field. Both fat and weak children could beat their athletic colleagues on *effort*. This made the run attractive to all.

Note that maximum safe heart rate is traditionally calculated as :

$$220 \text{ b.p.m. minus your age}$$

This is a good guide, but studies have yielded more accurate rates, such as by Miller in 1993 at Indiana University :

$$217 \text{ b.p.m. minus } (0.85 \times \text{your age})$$

This daily exercise regime had a profound effect on the children for the remainder of the day. Academic capabilities were enhanced, as demonstrated when the school finished 1st worldwide in the science part of the International TIMSS test in 1999. But social behaviour was significantly improved also, along with attentiveness during lessons. And finally, the weight of 97% of the children normalised to healthy levels.

Regular vigorous exercise necessarily improves cardiovascular health, increasing lung and heart capacities, and lowering both blood pressure and resting heart rate. The autopsy of Clarence DeMar, runner of some 1,000 or so races, revealed enlarged arteries. The demands of many long distance races made them more efficient at transporting substantial volumes of blood around his body. Exercise also helps your body regulate fuel better, and can aid weight loss for the obese, although it is important to stress that exercise alone cannot achieve consistent weight losses. The immune system is likewise strengthened.

But there are also changes to the brain. Sustained anaerobic exercise, such as sprinting, where there is not enough time to transport oxygen to the muscles to support the workload, has been shown to improve the efficiency of blood glucose transport, and hence improve the effectiveness of insulin.

It is generally well known that endorphins are released during exercise, making us feel happy and relaxed. Derived from the combination of the words endogenous (meaning internally generated) and morphine, their release from within is like morphine administered externally. They are of course a little addictive, hence the "runners high". But the elevated mood, coupled with the distractive effect of exercise can break negative trains of thought. I can personally testify to this effect, returning from 3 hours of football (soccer) to a matter that was troubling me beforehand, only to find that I could see the problem in a totally different light. In one sense, deeply engrossing exercise is a form of meditation – you arrest the chatter in your mind as you focus on a single activity.

In addition to the feel good factor of exercise, recent research has shown that it can invoke neurogenesis – literally the creation of new neurons in the brain. These neuronal stem cells mostly appear in the hippocampus. [SP] They migrate to the dentate gyrus, a part of the hippocampus involved in receptivity to new experiences in life. When you exercise, you literally become more receptive to what is around you. What might have looked ordinary to you before becomes more novel, and you start embracing all and sundry. When you respond to this receptivity, and engage with the world more, the new neurons are liable to stick around. They are serving their purpose so justify their new existence. Exercise and engagement in the world is a virtuous circle.

Research has shown in rats that this neurogenesis only takes place when the exercise is performed voluntarily. [PM] Expressed conversely, rats forced to exercise under duress are on the defensive, and such a state of mind and body, even that of a rat, has a bearing on the effects of the exercise. When the sympathetic nervous system is engaged in a defensive stance, energies are focused on the negative. When exercise is voluntary, the rats happily trundle around their wheels, no longer on the defensive. This appears to enable neurogenesis.

If a prospering hippocampus makes engagement with the world an easy and natural matter, then consider the polar opposite – a shrivelled up hippocampus. It is no surprise that the hippocampus in both old and depressed people is often found to be reduced in size. The American Physiological Society (APS) Journal (18 Nov 2008) reported that exercise arrests the decline in neurogenesis in the aged. Research in 2005 by Bjornebekk, Mathe and Brene at the Karolinska Institute in Stockholm yielded a paper with the self explanatory title "The anti-depressant effect of running is associated with increased hippocampal cell proliferation."

My own simplistic viewpoint on this matter is that vigorous exercise has traditionally been the consequence of a hunt for food, and that when repeatedly engaged in hunting, the mind needs to be sharply aware of its environment. Catching any slight movement seen in the corner of the eye would be of great benefit when stalking prey. A receptiveness to the environment for navigation would also be of great value. To this end, it is probably no surprise that hippocampus growth is also accompanied by improved memory (from the same APS Journal edition).

Note also that exposure to novel situations also invokes neurogenesis. [HM] Exercise not only instigates neurogenesis, but the goal of the neurogenesis is to be more receptive to novelty then invokes further neurogenesis. Vitality breeds vitality.

The personality trait that has been labelled Attention Deficit Hyperactivity Disorder (ADHD) runs in my family. I have been blessed with the pros and cons of ADHD, allowing my mind to jump between seemingly unrelated ideas, linking them together. It also allows me to hyperfocus, as I do when I write, or when I play the Chinese game of Go. But ADHD is also a source of frustration to others, where my regular inability to pay attention to what they have to say without interrupting is hard for many to cope with. It appears that high levels of exercise affects the Locus Coeruleus, thereby making the ADHD brain less likely to act out of proportion to a situation, thereby reducing interruptions. The over active cerebellum in the ADHD type, which often causes fidgeting in children, is also calmed down by exercise. fMRI scans of ADHD brains show that exercise can improve the ability of the reward centre (Nucleus Accumbens) to inform the prefrontal cortex that something is interesting enough to pay attention to. [SP] It may be no coincidence that movement and attention share common ground in the brain.

There appears to be a very welcome phenomenon arising from very strenuous exercise for those (like myself) who have suffered panic attacks. The resulting elevated heart-rate is similar to that experienced during a panic attack. However, because of the context – the exercise that is causing the elevation – and because of the endorphin saturated state, the high-heart rate now has a positive association. The subconscious can stop labelling elevated heart-rates as a cause for concern. [SP]

It was a little surprising for me to learn that general fitness rather than the specific type of exercises you undertake is better correlated with good health. [SP] It is more important for your health that the exercise you undertake maintains a good level of fitness now, than what you did in your younger years. In other words, the effects of a life time of inactivity appears to be readily reversible. The long term fit take only about 2 days of exercise to recover after 2 weeks of inactivity, whereas the unfit take much longer, and are likely to suffer days of aching muscles before they get there.

It appears that a single good aerobic workout can lower blood pressure for nearly 24 hours. Yet even walking is extremely good for you. Lacking the percussive impact of running or running based sports such as tennis, walking has been described as the perfect exercise. Even a long 3 m.p.h. walk can raise metabolism by more than a factor of three. [SP] If you can exercise in your job, all the better – research showed that risk of Cardiovascular Heart Disease (CHD) was halved in heavy labouring workers compared to their sedentary counterparts. [SP] There is also a strong case for replacing surgery with an exercise programme for CHD sufferers. [SP] Part of the problem with surgery is the damaging effects of anaesthetics and possible exposure to bacteria and viruses.

I have so far discussed dynamic physical exercise. Disciplines such as yoga are more concerned with awareness of your body, and the relationship between your body and your mind. Although this Indian practice extends into spiritual matters, for many it provides a calming form of exercise that improves muscle tone and posture. A principle benefit of improved posture is relief from internal organ compression that many suffer with. It would especially benefit myself as I am often to be found hunched over my keyboard. Compressed organs necessarily fail to operate optimally. Yoga is also deeply concerned with breathing. Most of us do not breathe properly, in particular failing to breathe deeply enough.

I always misunderstood what shallow and deep breathing meant. Like many others, I guess, I assumed that it referred to the intensity and duration of our breaths. But deep breathing means to breath deeper – lower – down the torso, around our stomach area. This expands your lungs sideways, as this is the way they are meant to move. It is hard to learn this type of breathing, but worth the effort. The key aim is to fill all areas of your lungs with oxygen. Note that it is also crucial that wherever possible, the inward breath should be through your nostrils. It increases the efficiency of oxygen uptake, and results in a better breathing rhythm than through the mouth. The nostrils warm and filter the air, and the sinuses using nitric oxide to kill bacteria. If you develop the habit of mouth breathing, this can carry forward to night time, and can result in snoring or sleep apnea.

Chapter Fourteen

Injury and illness

Whilst exercise brings many benefits, there are downsides. The more strenuous the activity, the more likely you are to eventually sustain an injury. One of the downsides of the release of endorphins and adrenaline during exercise is that it numbs pain. [SP] I remember playing my first game of Sunday League football (soccer) as an outfield player at the ripe age of 39. I had been a goalkeeper until then, and struggled to coordinate with my fellow players, (as I still do in fact), with the net effect that I collided heavily with a fellow defender. I got badly winded in the process, but wanted to return to the pitch afterwards. I am glad that I did not since the dull pain in my side from the collision was in fact the heavily suppressed symptoms of broken ribs. A few hours later, the simple matter of driving my car was exquisite agony.

Not only does this pain suppression initially blind us to the reality of an injury, but our mind is also heavily focused on the exercise itself, so we tend to be reluctant to suddenly stop. Many a time have I continued to play and thereby aggravated what would otherwise have been a minor injury. By the way, the ribs took an agonizing 5 months to heal – an X-ray after 3 months stilled showed a visible fracture in one rib.

There are mixed opinions on how to minimize the likelihood of injury. Whilst it is universally accepted that you should gradually warm up, the benefits of stretching *before* exercise is a subject of much debate. A study of 1,538 Army Recruits at the Kapooka Health Centre in New South Wales in Australia found that stretching during pre-exercise warm ups had no tangible effect on injury avoidance. Stretching after exercise was shown to be effective, and it is likely that it does so by releasing some of the lactic acid that is accumulated in muscles during exercise. But other studies have shown that stretching before exercise *is* beneficial. My contribution to this is to strongly suggest that any pre-exercise stretching be performed *after* you have warmed up. The change in muscle state effected by a warm up is akin to the change in a stick of gum after a minute of chewing – you cannot snap a chewed piece of gum. What has always puzzled me, however, is that animals neither warm up nor stretch before sprinting to catch prey. For a big cat to sustain an injury would leave it extremely prone to attack, yet this appears to be a rare event.

The consequences for humans of injury are generally much less serious, but the point is that there are consequences. If we are unable to go to work, we are in a sense marginalised – taken out of the mainstream of life. So we lose some social contact, and maybe a loss of self-esteem because we are no longer pulling our weight at work. Sidelined by injury also means that we no longer receive the health benefits of exercise, and may comfort eat to compensate. With reduced calorific needs, this can readily result in weight gain. Stepping off the treadmill of life can bring about a cascade of problems in addition to the injury itself.

This is the case not just for injuries of course. Those who suffer with depression, for example, are predisposed to engage less and less with life, thereby increasing the isolation and the depression. Very much a vicious cycle. Whether it be through injury or illness, the loss of energy also results in a growing failure to keep on top of household chores, at least for those who live alone. The ensuing untidiness can cause upset, lowering a sense of harmony in our surroundings, and aggravating the depression further.

There are two points I want to make here. First that it is important to recognise that your decline in vitality can adversely affect the state of your house, trivial though that may sound. But much deeper is that you can also struggle to understand the cascading effect of the marginalisation injury or illness can bring. And your friends and family can often fail to appreciate your isolation. I have personally experienced this, with tension headaches since 1994 that eventually forced me to leave full time work in 2001. Over the subsequent years, it became a source of great frustration that the longer I experienced the debilitating effects of daily headaches, and therefore the more I wanted to explain my incapacity, the less that friends and family wanted to hear about them. I understand why, but it is still hard to deal with, since you end up coping in isolation. And one of the problems that then rears its head is that you have too much time to dwell on the isolating injury or illness. For many illnesses, especially those of mental origin, this serves not only to amplify and reinforce the illness, but also means that more time is spent in a negative mindset. Distraction from the illness with positive activities stops the illness ruling us, and also reminds the body that we want to be back doing things.

A large part of my investigations for this book was concerned with the tackling of this problem of isolation and withdrawal of support. Of strengthening mental resolve so that you can not only cope better, but also handle the lack of empathy and support without holding a grudge. Most of us are far too busy to have to listen to repeated stories of ill health from those around us. I very much know this because I have a friend who suffers headaches and I rarely remember to ask him about them.

It is worth noting that our sense of self, which gives us an awareness of our suffering, often serves to compound the suffering. Surprising though it may seem, animals can actually get depressed. Depression is initially simply a coping mechanism. A stranded animal may become depressed in order to preserve its resources until its mother finds it. But the difference between an animal and a human is that the animal does not mull on the state of depression as we do. It simply does not have the higher brain functions that allow us to *observe* the depressed state. And because we *can* observe, we start to let the depression affect our self esteem, which can enflame the depressive state beyond its initial purpose.

In summary, do not let marginalising matters *control* your life. Do not let your plight define you. Work around the problem. Years ago, I remember a friend in Portsmouth, England telling me about a building site accident that left him paralysed from the waist down at the tender age of 19. He said that it was the best thing that could ever have happened to him, since he discovered that he was an excellent wheelchair basketball player. And tennis player. He travelled the world, playing in International tournaments, even meeting his beautiful able-bodied wife-to-be at the German Open Wheelchair Tennis tournament. He was a very upbeat guy, yet the loss of feeling in both legs at such a young age could easily have driven him to a life of miserable self-pity. I used to enjoy rallying with him on the tennis court, his technique being better than mine, in spite of the constraint of the wheelchair.

The human brain generally works automatically around losses. We may be devastated when our girlfriend leaves us, but a few months later we are likely to be back to normal health. Some people do dwell on their losses, but most of us get over setbacks. Research has shown that even when hearing is lost, the brain compensates by using the auditory cortex for enhanced peripheral vision. [PM] This of course makes evolutionary sense, allowing the hard of hearing to see potential danger more readily at the fringes of their vision. The visual cortex takes up around a third of the human brain, so it is no surprise that loss of sight results in a cannibalising of this neuronal real estate not only by hearing but also by high level functions such as verbal memory. [PM] The enhancement to hearing is equivalent to improved peripheral visual, in the form of an increased sensitivity to sounds at quiet levels.

Note that much of the indoctrinating effects of the medical profession, along with the pharmaceutical industry, concerns our attitude towards pain and discomfort. If we get a headache, we automatically seek to anaesthetise it, to push it away. Many so-called primitive tribes, and philosophies like Buddhism, have a more pragmatic and intelligent view of pain and discomfort. They believe that pain and suffering are an integral part of the human condition, and that we should listen to what the pains are telling us, rather than blind ourselves to them. This may be hard to grasp, but an example may help see the value in this. Next time you have diarrhoea, do not automatically take a tablet to put a hold on your evacuations. The whole point is that the body *needs* to flush out what it sees as unwanted. My father used to bury his head under a towel above

121

a bowl of steaming hot water in order to flush out a cold. Symptoms are often both a valuable form of healing, and of communication that healing is taking place, yet we often do not accept them as part of life and as a sign of an active immune system.

Just as injury and depression can marginalise us, so too can illnesses. But many illnesses are simply a result of stresses and imbalances in the body. And also often a consequence of the wrong kind of thinking. These are termed 'Functional Illness', as opposed to the 'Organic illnesses' that have a defined pathology. [SI] Chronic Fatigue Syndrome (CFS), Irritable Bowel Syndrome (IBS) and Fibromyalgia are all examples of functional illnesses (FI's). They have no basis in viral or bacterial invasion, nor internal organ or biochemical failures. They are in essence, expressions of disharmony or imbalance. My tension headaches are most likely to be a combination of poor posture causing tightness in my neck, and an expression of chronic anxiety – my mind is on the defensive by default, using the headaches to hold me back from situations that have in the past been uncomfortable. At least, that is how I understand them.

Whilst functional illnesses have no definite pathology, they are generally as tangible and debilitating as organic illnesses. In many cases, they even mimic organic illnesses, which makes their diagnosis very difficult. This in turn can result in the misdiagnosis of organic illnesses. The majority for those who visit their doctor are likely to do so with functional illnesses. [SI] This is especially so for anxious people – those prone to mental stress. This is unlikely to be a recent phenomenon, although the intensity of modern working life may well have seen a rise in functional illnesses. Stresses and demands of daily life can be so overwhelming that it can literally make us ill. I'll describe ways to help avoid functional illnesses in the remaining chapters.

The accumulated effect of too much anger can manifest as heart, stomach and colon problems, too much sadness can manifest as problems in the oesophagus, and excessive fear as neck and back muscles pains. [SI] Fear is of course the underlying emotion of anxiety, meaning that chronic anxiety can indeed result in chronic headaches, for example. A profound difficulty with functional illnesses that become chronic is that the condition can disassociate from the cause. You may tense your neck muscle when you get anxious, but do this often enough and the neck muscle will hold onto the tension in the absence of the anxiety. I have personally often woken from blissful sleep with an intense headache, paradoxical and strange though this may seem.

To quote Freud :

"The symptom may have originally had a function, but the original reason for it has long gone, so it continues to function as an outlaw, a foreign body which keeps up a constant succession of stimuli and reactions in the tissue in which it is embedded."

Many functional illnesses also appear to be be the result of unexpressed emotions or traumas. [SI] There is reason why we get emotional of course, but a failure to express the emotion, trapping it internally, is detrimental to your health. There is, of course, a fine line between emotional suppression and emotional over expression. If something angers us, it is as bad to suppress the anger as it is to let it become full blown. Instead, we need to find out why we are angry and see that we need not be angry. To diffuse the situation.

For example, you may have a nagging thought in the back of your mind that you need to get a problem with your car fixed. This will create a little anxiety and an unsettled feeling. You should not suppress the nag or it will keep eating away at you, and your car will remain unfixed. You should take action – let the emotion coerce you into getting the car fixed. Suppressed emotions can result in headaches, tension and constipation, and excessive expressing of emotions can result in diarrhoea, inflammation and even vomiting. [SI]

In a general sense, health is the capacity to live life, unhampered by injury, illness or other physical and mental constraints. By this definition, we can compromise our health, albeit very slightly, by engaging in petty negatives, such as holding a grudge against someone else. The mere act of holding onto the grudge is a hampering one. A focus on retribution for

123

a past event detracts from our ability to live in the present – to live life in the now. An accumulation of negatives moves us away from living and steers us towards illness instead.

The stress of modern life also moves us away from health. But it is also prudent to point out that there are in essence two types of stress. Positive stress is where you push yourself in order to achieve more. It is often in a single direction, and has tangible rewards. Even for those who suffer psychological problems, pushing themselves to achieve, and becoming very tired as a consequence, is apparently more beneficial than damaging. This often results in a tiredness that is accompanied by a satisfied glow of achievement.

However, when we talk of stress, we are normally referring to negative stress, where we are pushed and pulled in multiple directions. This equates very well with material stress, where the shearing effect on physical objects that can literally tear them apart. Negative stress can also mean overload, where too much is happening for us to cope – too many simultaneous demands. Frequently, work, family and social forces set up obligations that create such negative stress – obligations that we cannot readily ignore. However, we can take action that minimises the opportunity for such negative stress.

First, we can simplify our lives by pruning out unnecessary commitments. We rarely recognise that we are as guilty in overloading ourselves as others are in adding to our burdens. For example, too many social events at weekends mean that chores are rushed and become burdensome. You are less likely to relax if you are always busy. Second, we can aim to single-task wherever possible. When writing this book, the less I interleaved that writing with other tasks, the better rhythm I got, and the greater my productivity. Single-tasking better suits the majority of us – chopping and changing carries with it natural inefficiencies

In addition to simplifying your life, it is wise to avoid negative people if you can – those who dwell on negative matters, complaining and criticising too often. They can both drain you and turn your mental focus to negative matters, creating a mind-state that attracts more negativity.

There is another vital technique that you can learn that will reduce the number of your obligations. This is the simple expedient of learning to say 'no' to demands placed upon you. By this of course I do not mean a belligerent blanket refusal to do anything for others, but to pick and choose, where you can, what you commit to. It is unwise to agree to do something for someone reluctantly, whilst also overloaded with other demands. My teacher sister, for example, feels an obligation to attend every each and extra curricula activity. By accepting only those that suit her agenda and interests, she attends in a better spirit, and is paradoxically likely to be appreciated more. By always agreeing to requests from others, they are more likely to take you for granted. By picking and choosing, they will value you for the ones you do agree to.

This concept is an example of psychotherapy, whose techniques can help expose and release the trapped emotions that can cause functional illnesses, and retrain us away from habits that fail to serve us well. There will be more on this later in the book. Meanwhile, exercise can alleviate many of the symptoms of stress, and relaxation can help to both calm and reset you mind and body.

Many functional illnesses result from bad habits. Habits that once served us well when young, but now cause us problems as adults. It is hard to both recognise and correct such habits. One man who had a recurring problem with sore throats was a certain F. M. Alexander, and the story of how he determined that this was the result of a bad habit and what he did to correct it is the subject of a later chapter.

Chapter Fifteen

Rest and relaxation

Modern society does not particularly value rest and relaxation. It often tends to equate it with laziness. But it is actually a vital component of good health. Part of the problem is that many of us neither do not know nor have never been told how to properly relax. It is assumed that being slumped in front of the television is relaxation. In a sense it is, as we rest our bodies, but a great deal of TV is concerned with maintaining our attention, so it is replete with devices that support this, with rapid scene changes, and regular bouts of high drama. The 'relaxing' habit of TV is often more a scene of mental bombardment. Much better to strap a pair of headphones on and escape with some 1970's Camel, where the music will flow over and calm you, rather than control your attention. Paradoxically, going for a gentle walk is also very relaxing, the rhythm of arm and leg movements working in sympathy with similarly paced rhythms in the brain.

One key benefit of rest and relaxation, when we do it right, is that we pause from our engagement with the world. We step off the gas and start to restore some balance to our over stimulated minds and bodies. However, be wary of taking too much rest, since inactivity can become established as a norm. A balance between work, rest and play is key.

One of the best expressions of relaxation is laughter, and this can be more readily at hand if you adopt the twin faceted philosophy of not taking life or yourself too seriously. I have been guilty of excessive seriousness, but now look for opportunities to used my new ever so slightly anti-serious approach to life to defuse tense situations and laugh if possible. Laughing when things go wrong is a great way of seeing them in a better perspective.

One of my most favoured relaxations is to lie in the sun with a good book. Bright, hot sunny days empower me as much as grey days can depress me. We are, however, all warned against 'unprotected' exposure to the sun. Except that this is yet another example of flawed guidance. [TT] In the decades following the time in the 1970's when Australians were first strongly advised to start covering themselves with sun tan lotion, skin cancers have proliferated. In reality, the only significant danger of sun exposure is excess that burns the skin. But even here, the damage is often just temporary soreness and some peeling skin. In extreme cases, sunburn can lead to cancer in the form of basal and squamos cell carcinomas, but even these are relatively easy to deal with.

The tough skin cancers – the melanomas – tend to appear on the parts of the skin that are *not* exposed to the sun. They appear to be instigated not by an excess exposure to the sun but by the converse – an overall lack of sun on skin, which leads to a lack of Vitamin D. This vitamin can only be produced by the body as a result of high elevation sunrays striking the skin.

Most sun-blocking lotions only block out UVB rays from the sun, and are poor at blocking UVA rays. Yet UVA makes up over 90% of all ultraviolet radiation from the sun. If you were to choose between UVA and UVB rays, you should prefer to block the former much more than the latter, because UVA rays are responsible for the more deadly skin cancers.[PP] Additionally, the UVB rays are responsible for the synthesis of Vitamin D! The application of sun block may well delay the UVB induced burning, but it effectively destroys the vital UVB production of Vitamin D. Because the lotion blocks burning, it thereby removes the signal – red and sore skin – that our bodies have normally used to inform us that we have been out in the sun too long. So we stay out in the sun longer, and absorb too much UVA radiation, thereby incurring a greater risk of cancers. But the lack of burning also means that we build up a natural tan – a natural protection against UVA rays – much more slowly, and hence still need sun tan lotion the next time. Note that it is not the sun striking our skin that directly creates the tan. Cells in our skin release melanin as a form of pigment. The tan is there to protect us against excessive UVA radiation.

In summary, it is much better to gradually acclimatise to the sun without lotion, building up a natural tan to protect you for longer and longer each day. Anecdotal it may be, but my mother diligently avoided the sun all the time that I can remember, yet was inflicted with, and died a slow death from skin melanoma. And to drive the point home further that it is the *lack* of sun that is the culprit in malignant skin melanomas, research indicates that these cancers are more prevalent the further away from the equator you go. Stopping the burning effect of the sun on your skin, and thereby allowing more damaging UVA rays in is akin to applying pain relief to an injury and continuing to exercise. The Michael and Mary Eades book "Protein Power life-plan" covers the effects of the sun in enormous detail, although quite how such a subject found its way into a book on high protein dieting is unclear. [PP]

Meditation is a form of relaxation that has been practiced for thousands of years. It brings enormous benefits, not least its anti-stress effects, that must make it the gold star standard of relaxation techniques. In summary, it is largely concerned with a calming of the stream of chatter from our subconscious that inflicts us, mostly unknowingly, all day long.

You can become aware of this chatter right now if you have a moment to spare. Just stop reading, and close your eyes. Then simply observe what thoughts and ideas 'pop' into your head. You might initially feel that you are consciously generating them until you try to disengage from them. As you ignore one thought another will swiftly arrive to replace it. If you try to consciously think of nothing, you will find it maddeningly hard to do so.

And this is where meditation comes in. It teaches you how to disengage the 'chatterbox'. When you watch TV, you essentially do disengage your chatterbox, but you also replace it with the 'gogglebox'. When the chatterbox or gogglebox are arresting your attention, you are not truly relaxed. After practice, meditation can help you achieve a relaxation that becomes a calmness free from arresting thoughts or interrupts. It can be deeply profound in its calming effect. With enough meditation experience, this calming effect can start to transfer to stressful life situations, helping you cope with them better.

There are many forms of meditation, and the mystique surrounding them tends to make most people regard them as an alien activity performed only by Buddhist monks sitting in the lotus position in a monastery. This really is a shame, since it is in fact most accessible to all, and indeed is an activity we all engage in unknowingly from time to time. When you pause to smell a flower, for that moment, you are absorbed in that smell. Nothing else exists. Your chatterbox briefly pauses as you live in that short moment. That this is a meditative state maybe best supported by the fact that many meditations involve an absorption in the beauty of a simple object, such as the flame of a candle. If you can, I recommend that you read up more about this subject, and give it a try. I meditate each night for 10 to 15 minutes and have found it to be a natural relaxing part of each day. On one occasion in a Swedish shop called Ikea, I had been suffering with a particularly intrusive headache when I sat down to meditate. Right in the middle of the busy and noisy cafe! Five minutes of meditation on the noises around me saw my headache reduced by half.

The main thing about this arresting of mental chatter, is that we are dealing with an attentional problem. When we rest, we really do not want to have to *attend* to matters that our minds might conjure up. We are resting, and we should be able to find time to let these matters wait until later. But our subconscious wants to keep nagging us. By focusing attention away from the chatter to a passive target, we achieve calmness. What we pay attention to becomes our reality.

Research into this matter of attention and perceived reality is very revealing. When a constant sound was played into the ears of subjects, brain scans revealed high activity in the auditory cortex. But the same subjects receiving the same constant sound but told to concentrate on a task showed much reduced auditory cortex activity, as if the sound had been reduced. When conscious attention was moved away from the sound, the brain simply reduced its efforts at responding to it. [PB] I particularly like this comment by J. Krishnamurti :

"Attention is the most basic form of love. By paying attention we let ourselves be touched by life, and our hearts naturally become more open and engaged."

It may be that those afflicted with ADHD have a fluctuating capacity to love because of their attentional difficulties.

Compassionate meditation has become one of the best established forms of meditation. Unlike the calm meditation mentioned above, it is a more dynamic variation, with consciously chosen thoughts of compassion about people you know employed as the focus away from the stream of unconscious chatter. The idea here is to replace the neutrality of calmness with a more overtly positive construct. It requires much effort and persistence, and is quite hard at first. But eventually, not only can you hold loving and compassionate mental images and thoughts about your friends and family, but also, the people in your life who irritate or hurt you. The daily practice of compassionate meditation can eventually strengthen the left frontal cortex, weakening the right frontal cortex, the bringer of ill thoughts.

This may well sound idealistic because most of us are so caught up in life that we have no time to ourselves, let alone the luxury of compassionate meditation. But if you can create time, and sustain it for months or years, you will treat your fellow man, woman and child with an increasingly receptive manner, and move away from the very common perpetually defensive mindset. But most profound of all is that you will start seeing the world as less threatening, and actually raise your happiness set-point. [SH]

This set-point is the general level of happiness we settle down to after a big event, either positive or negative. It had long been assumed that our 'normal' level of happiness was pretty static in the long term. However, just as the brain has now been show to be much more neuroplastic (essentially meaning capable of rewiring itself) than previously imagined, emotional states that arise from the brain are also subject to change. Given enough desire and effort, we can become happier. And this subject gets its own chapter later.

I want to broach a highly sensitive subject now. I do so from a position of zero personal experience, but with enough confidence in what I have learnt to be convinced of the value of what I have to say. I am talking here of the use of Marijuana, (or Cannabis as it is alternatively known) as a legitimate relaxant. And the pivotal point here is that marijuana is much more than this. Research has shown it to be effective against cancer, glaucoma, multiple sclerosis, Tourettes syndrome, obsessive compulsive disorder, Chrons disease, depression and more. It enhances receptiveness, lowers aggression, and increases the appetite. (Hence the infamous 'munchies').

Until being caught up in the so called 'War on drugs', marijuana was regularly prescribed for health reasons. In his enlightening book "Junk Medicine", Theodore Dalrymple lays down a strong case against this phoney war, and against the common consensus that marijuana is a gateway drug, inevitably leading to heroin and cocaine use. [JM] His was no theoretical viewpoint. He had worked with so-called addicts in both prison and hospital for over a decade. He was able to see at first hand that even those who took heroin were able to endure the side effects of withdrawal without long term consequences. In many cases, the withdrawal was akin to a bout of influenza – uncomfortable but of finite duration and not life threatening. He believes that when 'addicts' are eventually seen by the medical profession, that they claim that they are too addicted to stop. He has seen, however, many addicts weaned off their drug with almost no side effects when administered a placebo saline solution in place of the methadone they were told they were being given. It is highly likely that governments benefit financially from this perpetual phoney war.

Whilst the basis of such a war is not directly relevant to this book, that it is being perpetuated for financial reasons does have a bearing. Marijuana is illegal in both the US and UK, with prison terms for growing it. This blanket ban stops the health benefits of marijuana reaching many people. A colleague of mine has suffered with the grim reality of 30+ years of depression. His illegal supply of marijuana is one of the few mechanisms he has found that can lift him into some kind of normal, healthy mental state, embracing life rather than being driven to tears by the state of his brain chemistry. Is it really right that he should be criminalized for using the health benefits of marijuana simply because some young people abuse this drug? If the abuse of a drug is a criteria for its ban, where does that place alcohol in the scheme of things?

The health and society damaging effects of alcohol are enormous in scale, but it is classified as safe. Drug experts in the UK placed both alcohol and tobacco ahead of marijuana in their own classifications (The Guardian and other Newspapers, 3rd November 2009), reflecting the reality of the impact of each drug, and very much at odds with the classification adopted by governments. And this in spite of the fact that the former advise the latter. It is of course true that alcohol used intelligently in small quantities can be a great relaxant, with much research endorsing the health benefits of red wine for example. But it appears to be far more addictive than the hard drugs. It is all too common for an occasional tipple to become a regular, focal point of the day, with larger quantities consumed as the years pass.

I had a serendipitous meeting with a lady in a coffee shop last weekend. She had been attentive to the conversation I was having with the owner. When she came over to sit with me, I discovered not only that she had aspergers syndrome – a mild, high functioning form of autism – but that she is actively helping others with aspergers, and was able to rapidly recognise that I too was somewhere along the autistic spectrum. I was aware that I came under the ADHD umbrella, but I was quite close, it seems, to being aspergic. Our conversation should have been videoed, as I suspect the rapport we immediately had, along with our mutual ability to interrupt each other would have been amusing to observe. You will recognise that I have sidetracked from my story now. I hope you allow me this, but one reason for doing so is to illustrate a feature of the semi-aspergic mind I have – the effortless capacity to forge links between anything and everything. It lets me link drugs to sleep, as you will shortly see.

Sleep is the ultimate form of relaxation. In reality, however, it is a lot more than this. It does supply physical rest, where the body is calmed down, but it is also time for the events of the day, along with their consequences to be pondered. If you had been working on a problem in the evening, the brain will continue to work on it overnight, which explains why we can awaken with what appear to be 'sudden' insights.

The onset and duration of sleep is largely governed by the pineal gland. Often referred to as our third eye, lying in the very centre of the brain, it has connections to the optic nerves, allowing it to be aware of night and day, and by virtue of the length of daylight hours, the season. It controls sleep patterns – the circadian rhythm – and in animals also controls seasonal breeding patterns.

The main product of the pineal gland is the hormone melatonin, which induces and sustains sleep. Marijuana has been shown to significantly enhance the effects of melatonin, hence explaining in part the relaxing effect of that drug. Until as recently as the 1980's, the pineal gland was mostly ignored, seen as an anomaly much like the appendix. This was in part because the levels of melatonin it secretes are minute, tricky to measure, and were originally deemed too tiny to be of importance. Russell Reiter was one of the key early melatonin researchers, and the more he researched this hormone, the more he recognised its importance.

Melatonin appears to be present in all animals, and has been so for billions of years without any change to its chemical structure. One fortuitous aspect of melatonin is that it is extremely easy to synthesise in a form that is chemically identical to that produced by the pineal gland. However, because it cannot be patented and exploited by Big Pharma, its benefits have been mostly suppressed. Or more pertinently, the value of melatonin to health has been poorly broadcast to the public. Whilst it is freely available in health food shops in the US, here in the UK it must be prescribed by doctors. This disparity is odd, but it appears that the defensive UK posture is based on the lack of long term research into its safety.

In his excellent book "Melatonin", Reiter describes the standard LD50 test used to explore safe levels of a drug. [ME] This test seeks to discover the level of a drug ingested by rats that would cause 50% of them to die. The test failed to complete for melatonin because the rats were incapable of consuming enough melatonin to reach the 50% fatality level. The level of melatonin they were administering had reached the equivalent of 50,000 times the normal human dosage. Compare this with the fatal overdose levels of aspirin and paracetamol, and it is readily apparent that on safety grounds, the UK ban for sale was on the wrong products. (There are many articles on the Internet that reveal quite how dangerous aspirin is, in spite of its acquired label of safety). Unlike the stomach pumping required for an overdose of many freely available drugs, an overdose of melatonin generally simply results in daytime drowsiness. Doses even as high as 1,000 mg have elicited only sleepiness, with no other apparent side effects.

Melatonin is taken to aid sleep not only for insomniacs, but also for the elderly, and as a jet lag aid in the airline industry. Until recent years, it had been assumed that you needed less sleep as you got older. This is partly true – teenagers need large amounts of sleep, but less so as they reach their twenties. But the tendency of the elderly to awaken prematurely, often at 4 or 5 am, and then to struggle to fall back to sleep because of the lack of circulating melatonin is actually damaging to health and alertness. They need the extra sleep that depleted levels of melatonin deprive them of. Slow release melatonin tablets taken at night can remedy this, allowing the elderly to sleep longer and hence awaken more refreshed and energised for the day. A normal dose of melatonin is around 1 mg, although seem to require 10 mg daily, whilst others happily operate on much less than 1mg .

If you feel uncomfortable taking melatonin supplements, you can elevate your own levels by taking daily exercise in bright sunlight for at least an hour, along with a reduced use of bright light levels in the few hours before sleep. If the sun does not shine, a Seasonal Affective Disorder (SAD) lamp can suffice.

Calcium is vital for the production of melatonin. Melatonin can also be obtained from some foods, oats being one of the richest sources. And whilst a carbohydrate, a small bowl of porridge for supper actually aids sleep enormously. A small quantity of carbohydrates prior to sleep, as long as high in glycemic index, can actually help you to relax. This effect used in conjunction with time-release melatonin can vastly improve sleep patterns.

Whilst I am principally discussing the impact of melatonin on sleep, it is so valuable a hormone that it is worth digressing and revealing more of the nature of this mostly ignored hormone. Melatonin differs in a number of ways from all other hormones, not least that it is produced in tiny amounts. Normally, the cells of our body have receptors in their walls for hormones. But there are no melatonin receptors – the melatonin is allowed to pass through the cell walls and make its way directly into the cell nucleus. It appears that the levels of melatonin finding their way into cell nuclei are correlated with cell life-spans. Tests on rats given elevated melatonin supplements in their diet lived up to a third longer. [ME]

In addition to its role in rest, melatonin triggers and enhances bodily repair processes. It is no surprise then that melatonin has been seen to boost the power of the immune system. Melatonin has, in effect, the opposite effect of adrenaline and cortisone, both of which bring us into an alert state and which put the immune system on hold. Indeed, stress lowers melatonin levels. Melatonin supplementation can compensate for the effects of stress. Surgery also has a weakening effect on the immune system. Administrating melatonin following surgery has been shown to accelerate immune system recovery. [ME]

Note that caffeine and the twin 'evils' of alcohol and tobacco also serve to deplete melatonin levels. Paradoxically, however, a little alcohol just before sleep can actually have the opposite effect, helping us slip into sleep more readily. Some pharmaceutical drugs, especially beta blockers, can damage sleep patterns, such is their effect on melatonin. If you must take these drugs, it is much better therefore to do so in the morning.

In its repair role, melatonin has been shown to be the most potent and versatile anti-oxidant. It also helps to regulate the heart-rate. Patients with hypertension had normalised heart-rates within one week of taking melatonin supplements. ME   There was indeed a correlation found between healthy hearts and naturally high melatonin levels. ME Melatonin can also prevent and reduce cancers, and works very well in concert with anti-cancer drugs. It also relieves premenstrual discomfort and the effects of the menopause. As if this were all not enough so far, melatonin can also assist in recovery from depression, and in the health of diabetics. Low melatonin levels were found in schizophrenics, manic depressives, diabetics, alcoholics, and those with Alzheimer's disease.

An afternoon nap can also allow you to catch up on a sleep debt – the Spanish siesta to avoid working in the hottest part of the day is a prudent idea. I have personally used afternoon naps to recover from many a bad night's sleep. But I have now cultivated a technique that lets me fall back to sleep more readily if and when I awaken early. The health gains from sleeping well are enormous, but sleep can be evasive.

No matter whatever else in your life might have under control, you essentially have no direct influence over your sleep. The more you seek to fall asleep, the more likely to are to stay awake. Sleep has to be allowed to 'happen'. And to facilitate this happening, I have now learnt to relax. I physically relax my body, clear my mind as if meditating, and, crucially, place no urgency or expectation on falling asleep. By simply lying in a calm, relaxed state, free from angst about the need for sleep, or energised by streams of thoughts, I invariably fall asleep, sooner or later, often awaking refreshed for the day ahead.

If I awake early, I do not curse the lack of sleep, but again lay relaxed. I stay relaxed for as long as it takes to fall back to sleep again, only arising when my sleep debt has been paid. True, I am extremely lucky to be self-employed and therefore have no fixed schedule, but do find that if I aim for the best night of sleep, I am normally repaid with amazing energy levels in the day that more than make up for any late rising.

Chapter Sixteen

Meaning in life

Good food, exercise and rest are key to optimum health, but these are all principally physical matters. It is time to move on to the mind, and how we engage in life. It is far from sufficient to be in good physical health, and, I would argue, more important that we are in good mental, emotional, social and spiritual health. Note that you do not have to be religious to fully embrace spiritual concepts – I refer here to the embracing of a deep meaning in life and the planet that goes beyond day to day matters.

A fundamental component of good mental health is to be occupied in ways that give you a sense of meaning in life. Much as we may complain about the need to work, it is often a cornerstone for our health. It allows us to channel our abilities and energies into tangible achievements that benefits both ourselves in the satisfaction of achievement and others in the delivery of goods or services. It also supplies us with money to finance our lives. The workplace supplies a community that is like an extension of family life, and maybe even a catalyst for a new family, since many meet their future partner there.

Work is often the core of life for many – it provides an ongoing sense of worth and meaning. I like to think of it as an anchor upon which our life can be tied. There is a danger to health, however, if we let work dominate too much. Not only in the obvious sense that we overload ourselves with stress, but that we lose balance. Work is no longer an anchor but the be-all and end-all of our lives. Putting all eggs in one basket is dangerous. Good health is all about balance, even though this might appear to be too obvious to need stating. But we can get blinded by job promotions and higher salaries and fail to see that we often absorb much of the extra money this brings on luxuries and over-eating to compensate for the stresses of the extra work load or responsibilities. Stress at work is not intrinsically bad for us. If you work hard in a positive direction, as already mentioned, then stress is good for you. But engage in a job with conflicting demands, or simply overload, and you can burn out.

The converse of a work-obsessed life is one spent in many diverse ways. The adage that 'Variety is the spice of life' is a sensible one. I would say that variety is fundamental to good health, and that a heavy domination of any one part of your life, whether it be work or even a hobby, can cause an unhealthy imbalance. But there are secondary benefits from greater variety in your life.

First, that the loss of any single aspect of you life is then less likely to be damaging. The loss of one of many things you engage in is less unbalancing. If work dominates, then the loss of your job will be devastating, but if work is part of a rich and varied existence, you will cope better in the limbo period before finding new work.

Second, a life of variety fosters a sense of flexibility – as life changes, you go with the flow. Lose your job, and you are much more capable of finding a job in a different discipline than if your life was very limited.

One avenue of variety is to engage in hobbies. The Chinese game of Go has been a core part of my life, and I am suitably indebted to my brother for introducing the game to me in 1990. My Go playing friends are some of the most interesting people I know, people I may never otherwise have met. Likewise, soccer and tennis have provided me with great health benefits and hundreds of acquaintances. Both Go and sport also serve to detach my mind from daily routines, from worries and woes.

Religion of course provides vast numbers of people with a deep sense of meaning in their lives, and moral guidance to boot. Not only can deep faith become central to your life, but it can become resiliently so. Religion is a source of meaning that transcends and is impervious to all that might happen to us in our lives. You only have to witness those praying in the aftermath of the 2004 Indonesian Tsunami to be reminded of this resilience of faith. That religions are open to, and receive much criticism, is rarely enough to undermine them. Nor does criticism negate the value of religions. Even if a religion is perhaps based upon delusional thinking, this thinking is overtly optimistic, and as such very healthy. And if you are not religious, and mock delusion based optimism, then you will probably not like to be informed that optimistic people are more delusional about reality than pessimists, and generally healthier as a consequence. Their rose tinted glasses delude them in to seeing things better than they often actually are.

To convert your hobby or interest into a job is in a sense the ultimately desirable way to go to work. A vocation, no less. Again, be wary that it might limit your flexibility and variety in life. But there is another aspect to hobbies that can provide the kind of long-term gains that work supplies. To have dreams and plans, and to fulfil them is a great way to improve vitality. In my view, living out a dream is more exciting than any job could be.

One of my dreams was to publish a book on the Chinese game of Go. I felt in my bones that I could deliver a book that would fill a niche in the burgeoning Go book marketplace. But discovered, as many others also do, that many obstacles can litter the path. At the very outset I was told by the British Go Association book-seller that it was not worth publishing because there were already too many books on the market (he subsequently stocked and sold a number of my books). And there is the additional highly relevant fact that I am a considerably weaker Go player than the authors of *all* existing Go books. Bar none.

However, I skirted around these and other problems, believing in the fun and feasibility of what I was doing. I was taking a risk, living in a society that has become risk adverse. Taking risks is all part and parcel of richness and variety in life. The ensuing vitality it gives you has a very positive effect on your health. Being creative is likewise a zest giving part of life.

When problems presented themselves with the book, I worked around them, rather than give in. If you can see problems as challenges, skirt around them, and even learn from them, then you can grow stronger in the face of future challenges.

I now have three Go books self-published on Amazon. When pursuing a dream, it is key to remember that achieving the dream is only a part of the deal. The anticipation and journey along the way represent the vital parts of a dream – be wary that achieving a dream can occasionally be anti-climatic. [15]

Vital to life and health are of course your partner, friends and family. They also supply a sense of meaning and perspective in your life, lifting you when it is needed and grounding you when you get too full of yourself. A happy marriage is also a key indicator of good health, but it is actually better to be single than to struggle with a failing relationship. Humans are social people, gaining many benefits from group synergy. But we are all very different, and social cohesion can be very demanding at times. If you fail too far or too often to adhere to social rules, you can be ostracised, and this is extremely damaging for your health.

I have noticed that there is sadly an asymmetry with regard to social obligations and niceties. It is all too easy for the odd ill-thought-out comment or misdeed to result in years of mistreatment, as people can harbour a deep and persistent grudge against you. Slight disagreements in outlook can keep family members at loggerheads with each other for years. Recognise how very much humans are different from each other, even within a family, and give your fellow man or woman some slack in order to get on better with those around you.

One consequence of modern social structures, and modern life in general, is that more and more of us suffer with loneliness. I visit coffee shops each day to escape the necessary solitude of writing. Fortunately, I enjoy my own company a lot, and rarely feel lonely. I suspect this is a manifestation of the autistic side of my personality. But for many people on their own, and especially the old, loneliness is a big problem. Research by Professor John Cacioppo of the University of Chicago has revealed a swathe of health issues arising from social isolation. There is a greater resistance to blood flow, higher morning stress levels, higher levels of depression, a degradation in the quality of sleep (probably because of lowered melatonin levels), and accelerated Alzheimer's disease.

But these are not irreversible, as I recently learnt from a neighbour. This sweet and friendly 87 year old regularly took in parcels for me when I was out. Her son visited every day, bringing all her meals and doing all her washing. He too was a genuinely nice man. She was essentially house bound, with books, the TV and the radio her principle friends. She seemed to enjoy the short chats with me when I collected my parcels. On one occasion, I sat with her indoors, showing her some Wedding photos I had taken. I happened to notice then how much she repeated herself.

One day recently, I learnt from her son that her legs could no longer carry her around her house, and that she had to be taken into hospital for investigation. Early in her stay, I visited her, and repeatedly she said how good the hospital food was. Casting aside the possibility that she might now also be delusional, I did sense a greater energy. And there was one telling thing she said regarding her welfare. She now had so many visitors that she had no time to watch her 'soaps'. For someone who relished a good chat, this was good news.

Just a few weeks later, prior to her transfer to a private home, her son told me that her dementia was in decline. She repeated herself less, and was in much better grip of her mental faculties. She had been drawn back into the mainstream of life, engaging with a diversity of people, and regaining the vitality required to engage with them. You see, talking is one of the best exercises for the brain!

Chapter Seventeen

Happiness

When we have good health, eat well, exercise well, have a good job, a fabulous partner, healthy children, a great house, exciting hobbies, and no money worries, you would imagine that our lives would be blissfully content and happy. So why is it that many get this far and remain unhappy? And why is it that many others fall far short of such achievements and status, yet remain permanently happy and content with life?

Part of this is down to genetics, which can predispose some to a life of depression, and others to be happy regardless of circumstance. It is a harsh reality that some of us have a raw deal regarding our inherited happiness set-point. However, genetics is but one factor affecting our happiness and contentment, or there would be no point in me writing this chapter.

The human brain is very dynamic – very neuroplastic – so genetics guide us more than they dictate. You know yourself that your personality has changed since childhood, so you have already experienced nurture overriding nature. But we can affect much deeper changes to ourselves than we might imagine. Rather than allow social forces and random changes to sculpt who we are, we can choose the path we take.

As I studied the books I used for research, I cherry picked a set of concepts that I have adopted ever since in my own life, to change how I behave, and hopefully raise my happiness set point. One of these new concepts was to simply *try* to be happier. This is almost a taboo concept in the UK, I should add. The very idea of trying to be happier is generally greeted with much scepticism, the pervading belief being that the acquisition of a falsely happy persona is just downright stupid and annoying.

But there are two points here I want to cover. First that it is plain to my eyes that to be happy is a pretty unarguably positive thing to aim for. If achieving it involves a transition through simulated happiness, then so be it. To become athletic when initially weak must surely mean an interim period of small muscles sat atop a weak frame. But that is a sign of progress, not a cause for ridicule or abandonment of the fitness drive. Second, that a fundamental part of our difficulty in making changes in our attitude to life is that we have precious little education on the concept in school. The teaching of mental, emotional, social and spiritual growth, and of the setbacks that accompany them is only occasionally, and sporadically taught in schools. It appears that matters such as the methods of irrigation of land in an alien country, or stories of Kings and Queens from centuries past, are deemed more important than the teaching of ways to live more healthily. This baffles and frustrates me – fundamentals are bypassed in favour of detailed digressions into matters meaningless to most people's lives.

Rick Foster and Greg Higgs wanted to explore the concept of happiness in an empirical manner, and so travelled to various countries in search of the happiest person in each locale they visited. The summary of their findings in "How we choose to be happy" [HH] is not entirely predictable, and makes an interesting read as a consequence. Indeed, the number one habit of happy people appears to contradict the common consensus that happy people are just happy by nature. Foster and Higgs found that most very happy people actually make a conscious effort to be happy. They do indeed work on their happiness, and intentionally seek to take the happy route through life. Whatever happiness that was innate was seemingly not enough on its own to propel them to the high levels of happiness they have achieved in their lives. They had to keep working at it. Most of us do not even try to be happy in the first place!

They worked out what made them happy, and made that a key focus in their lives. When they did encounter problems and had bad experiences, they did not succumb to these negatives, but worked around them and eked out some positives. They used these undesirable events as teachers. And just as they steered around problems, they allowed life to guide them rather than forcing life to be at their beck and call – they stayed flexible, going with the flow, taking risks and embracing the spontaneous. Accompanying the flow was an awareness of the world around them, and a deeper appreciation of many facets of life that the rest of us take for granted. And from this flowed a natural tendency to give, as a thanks for all that they received. Not on a one for one basis, where a favour by one is returned by another. But a giving of goods or services from the heart, with no expectation of return.

And finally, Foster and Higgs learnt that very happy people tend to be very honest with themselves and others, and disciplined in their lives, taking responsibility for their actions. If they promise to do something, they will make sure it happens. If they make a mistake, they own up, and seek to make up for their failing. Whilst there are a number of social situations where honesty is a dangerous policy, the ongoing consequences of honesty is that you are true to yourself and others and can relax more. You have nothing to hide. This is one of the concepts that I have personally tried to adopt for many months now, and one that I really enjoy working at. Honesty is a key aspect of Taoism, as it works hand in hand in reducing the grip that the ego has on many of us, as you will learn later in the book.

Absent in these key findings was any mention of 'pleasure'. Most people readily confuse pleasure with happiness. And do so repeatedly, failing to heed the lessons of the past – that the fabulous new gadget in the post now will make them happy. Pleasure is transient. It is like the icing on the cake. The novelty of the gadget will wear off within a few days, and a restlessness will kick in until the next pleasure 'fix'. Happiness is, in a sense, an ongoing contentment with life. To be happy is much less a focus on things and events than it is an attitude that allows us to go with the flow, and enjoy anything and everything that might happen. We are not caught up in expectation. Happiness is in effect a by-product of the right attitude. The more we seek happiness, like sleep, it will elude us. Happiness is the 'glow' that comes from an ability to cope with whatever life brings, seeing beauty and fun wherever it might manifest. You only have to look at children to see this in action – they do not rely on pre-conceived ideas of what will make them happy to guide their behaviours, and so find happiness in many things.

I remember on one particularly wet Saturday afternoon that only seven of us turned up for our informal game of soccer in the local park. We were lucky enough to be challenged to a game by a group of children, all in their early teens. Until, that is, we realised how much more skilled they were than us. But what stuck in my memory most was the stark contrast in attitudes of the two teams. The children simply laughed more – finding late tackles and trick plays funny, whereas we adults had seen it all before and could no longer laugh. These children found exquisite pleasure in belly flopping into puddles. True, they would not be the ones to clean their muddy clothes, but they demonstrated spontaneous happiness. They were living in the moment, and were happy doing whatever, going with the flow. Imagine actually planning to go to the park to dive into puddles. Even children would not do it. And if they did plan to do so, they would not have enjoyed it as much. It was not so much that the puddle diving was pleasurable, but that the capacity to be spontaneous demonstrated a happy state of mind. A liberated mindset.

If you embark on an activity, and invest your future pleasure in that event, you are focusing on pleasure, and are not keeping a happy mindset. Seeking and expecting pleasure in a meal will fail to make you happy if the meal is not up to standard. And if the meal is great, then how do you sustain the pleasure when it is finished? A happy mindset is one that does indeed enjoy a good meal, and appreciate it more deeply also, but that does not cling to that pleasure.

As I mentioned earlier, a successful career and family life does not guarantee happiness. Success is not readily correlated with happiness. The right attitude, as you have seen, is correlated with happiness. Even those with lives impoverished by most standards can be happy by virtue of their attitude to life, making the most of their circumstances. But success coupled with the right attitude can indeed make for a really rich and fulfilling life. Just do not expect attainments themselves to make you happy.

Nor should you get caught up in material things. The British popular science journal, 'The New Scientist' explored the effect of phones, the Internet and computers on our lives (Issue 2739, Dec 2009). Daniel Goleman reported that our investment in these 'vital' components of modern life is taking us away from face-to-face contact and actually depressing us. These electronic devices are in effect enslaving us. You can get a sense of this when you observe exactly how often you check your email. Psychologist Tim Kasser of Knox College in Galesburg, Illinois, has shown that a focus on material things makes us less happy. It also lowers our self-esteem, and tends to make us seek material comparisons with others, investing our happiness in the superiority of the things we own to what others around us own. Indeed, any form of comparison is doomed to destabilise our health.

Addiction to these modern technologies, and especially to games consoles, damages our sense of autonomy and self competence. We are bound by the rules of a machine, and removed from interactions with humans. However, if we seek out just the *experiences* of modern technology, and do not allow ourselves to be *controlled* by these devices, then we are relatively free from their harms. And this leads to a key concept. Research has shown that we are much more likely to be happy by choosing experiences instead of material things. Much better to rent a few DVDs rather than 'own' one.

There is a neat mechanism you can employ to minimise the chance that material things will enslave you. Whilst the title of his inspiring book, "Infinite self : 33 Steps to reclaiming your inner power" is a bit suspect in my view, Stuart Wilde has a massive amount of wisdom to offer the reader. [IS] He says that it is best to see the material things in your life, including your house and car, as being *on loan* to you. This kind of thinking is very liberating, and you have seen that a key to happiness is a liberation from attachment. If your computer is seen as on loan by the world to you, as long as you respect this entitlement, then its grip on you is neutralised. To reinforce this 'loan' concept, just remember that you take no material things with you when you die.

Alas, modern life has indoctrinated many into the wrong kind of thinking. The focus on material things, and the inherent short-termism that this entails is no better illustrated than with the motor car. We are almost universally caught up in the 'need' to own a car, but fail to see the global and long term consequences. Until recently, that is, when the polluting effects of cars has become a hot topic. But this obsession with cars has caught up with us in many other ways, and this form of material possession has been hugely damaging to the quality of modern life. It is wirth detailing precisely how far cars have damaged our lifestyles.

It was not long before cars caused the scarring of the landscape, as more and more roads and motorways were built. The ability to drive became almost a mandate to drive. Home and work could now be separated not just by miles, but by tens of miles, making foot and cycle travel unfeasible, adding to the pollution, tiring out the commuter before they have started work, and effectively extending the length of the working day. The exhausted traveller is then less likely to have the time and energy for quality home life. Life balance is damaged. And the excessive travel can create farcical situations where someone living in Cardiff can be travelling to Bristol to work in the same type of job that sees a Bristol man travel to Cardiff. Likewise, shops are spread more thinly, with many large shops sited out of town, mostly inaccessible to those without transport.

The status of the car is also elevated ahead of that of the pedestrian. That a human in a polluting car so often has right of way over a non-polluting human crossing the road is madness if you are to really think about it. But when we get behind the wheel of a car, the car changes our behaviour. It corrupts us. Pedestrians are humans like us, but they move much more slowly and are relegated in importance in our eyes. So much so that most drivers will not indicate at a roundabout to inform a pedestrian of their intent. The pedestrian has to blindly wait before crossing, or guess by the angle of the wheels whether the car will exit the roundabout or not. The failure to indicate is actually a social failure on the part of the driver, but he is blinded to this by the empowering effect of the car. It is technically also a driving failure, although very few motorists know that the need to signal intent extends to *all* road users. When a pedestrian is trying to cross the road, he is indeed a road user. But we fail to embrace such concepts because we allow the power of the car, this material thing, to corrupt our humanity.

Children rarely walk or cycle to school now, and the roads get clogged with the morning and evening transport of these children to and from school. This has the additional effect of removing some vital exercise from their lives. And a brisk walk, as we have already seen, is likely to sharpen their minds at the start of the school day. There is an additional, much more pervasive and damaging impact of the car on children. The sheer volume of street bound cars, both parked and mobile, means that the majority of streets have become no-go areas for most children, at least here in the UK. This problem is exacerbated by a media driven neurotic level of concern about child abduction and abuse that pushes children indoors, where they are apt to engage in the services of electronic devices. They not only become couch potatoes, but fail to engage with neighbours. A barrier of misunderstanding and alienation has grown between children and adults, in part because of our obsession with cars. And this has a long term damaging effect, as childhood is left behind and the reality of the real world is thrust that much harder upon children as they become young adults.

The loss of social bonding between adults that the car has also damaged is part of an additional set of problems with modern life. Big Industry has indoctrinated us to be consumers, and to focus on material things ahead of people. Traditions and traditional values have been swamped into misuse by the influence of capitalist society. Traditional recipes and herbal treatments have been marginalised and disqualified by Big Food, Big Medicine and Big Pharma. The intensity of modern life, with its heavy pressures to "keep up with the Jones's", and to work long hours has driven us away from the subtle things in life. We no longer have the time nor inclination to stop, look and listen to the world around us. We are racing on, seeking ever bigger fixes in the form of things or events, forgetting even to properly rest.

The default focus of governments in the UK, US and beyond is the economy, with the long held view that the wealth of the nation is key to their happiness. Part of the reason for the selection of this criteria is very simple. It is easy to measure and thereby relatively easy to control. It is quantifiable. By contrast, even though ultimately more important than money, the happiness of the people is a matter of quality and therefore considerably harder to measure, and enormously hard to control or influence.

However, according to Michael Baum, the Professor Emeritus of Surgery at University College London, there are very good measures of happiness. oncology departments regularly use psychometric instruments to determine well being. This is of particular value when determining if the impact of a cancer treatment programme is likely to be too damaging to well being, and hence should be avoided. Treatment may extend the life of a sufferer a little, but the quality of the extended life may be too low to justify that treatment. And the difficulty of measurement did not stop the remote Himalayan country of Bhutan from making the happiness of the people its number one priority. Yes, Bhutan put happiness ahead of the economy. Ahead of money matters.

They are somehow able to measure 'Gross National Happiness', and use it to make decisions. Not only have they banned street advertising as a consequence, believing its influence to be too manipulative, but they also stopped smoking in public places, on the grounds that this would have a net positive effect on overall health and happiness. But my favourite story from this small country concerns the introduction of the first set of traffic lights at a roundabout previously controlled by a human who directed the traffic with hand signals. There was such an outcry that the higher cost human was reinstated. Quality of life usurped cost. Happiness took priority over money.

Bhutan has one of the lowest ratios of earnings between the rich and poor, this being a key indicator of the health of a population. [SL] In those countries with very high ratios, most people are patently aware that they are well down the income ladder, with many frequently falling into the dangerous game of making comparisons. And those at the top are rarely helped by their excess wealth, such high incomes making them defensive as they look down the income ladder to those below who are after their jobs. The greater the income equality, the fiercer they have to defend their status.

Sadly, in economy-driven countries, the focus often eventually becomes one of cost-cutting. It is like cutting off your nose to spite your face. Rarely are traffic wardens seen wandering the streets, their hours drastically reduced, so that cars are frequently parked in ways that obstruct pedestrians and blindsight other drivers. Local council budgets are cut so much that roads become degraded with potholes, damaging cars, which result in law suits against the councils that deplete their tight budgets further still.

Returning to more direct impacts on happiness, there is one form of pleasure that does appear to enhance happiness. Laughter. And the rib bruising variety is wonderfully invigorating for both the soul and the immune system. Laughter follows the cue to not take life too seriously. If we laugh enough, the body moves away from a defensive posture to a life embracing one. My theory is that if you can laugh, then this tells your body that the environment is safe, so it can activate the parasympathetic nervous system to put us into a state of rest and repair.

If you choose to adopt any of the happiness-promoting ideas presented here, such as a happiness focused attitude, then it is crucial that you remember the pitfalls that can blight such an adoption. You must persevere, and be happy! And one final word on happiness. A happy, fun, enthusiastic outlook on life has been shown to result in a reduced chance of heart-attack or stroke (2010 European Heart Journal).

Chapter Eighteen
Force of habit

F. M. Alexander was an actor, and the sore throats he periodically suffered from badly affected his acting. [US] His doctor was at a loss at to the cause, so suggested periods of rest. When these failed to effect a cure, Alexander did some thinking. He noticed that lengthy periods of chatting to friends never resulted in sore throats, so he wondered exactly what he was doing differently when acting. Alexander was subsequently able to determine that his posture was causing his sore throats, using mirrors to diligently observe how he held himself differently when acting and when chatting. Now here is a matter that bemuses and amazes me – he observed his posture not for minutes, but for months. This demonstrates a fantastic and fanatical degree of patience.

These sustained observations appeared necessary because of the subtle nature of what he was investigating. Early on, he determined that his posture differed markedly when acting to that when casually chatting. He saw that his acting posture caused a compression of his larynx, that ultimately caused his throat to become sore. It was when he tried to correct it, however, that he had the greatest difficulties. As soon as he tried to change his posture *and* also to act, his posture reverted back to the faulty position. But he was, as I have said, a very patient man, eventually able to develop a technique for making the required postural change. He would repeatedly start acting, and each time simply *think* about the new posture, without adopting it. This would then bring the new posture into clear focus. Eventually, after repeated visualisations, he would apply the new posture, and start the change process, his mind now familiar with the new concept and therefore more accepting of it.

Key to his observations was that the intellectual value in a new way of doing something initially holds little sway against existing habits, *even when those existing habits have not served us well*. We repeatedly underestimate the control our habits have over us. One of the obvious reasons that a new habit struggles to replace an existing one is that the old and new behaviours exist and operate in different parts of the brain. The existing habit is run on autopilot by the subconscious, and the new behaviour that we want to become a habit, labours away in the slow conscious mind. Remember when you were learning to drive a manual car – how long it took to find the biting point, and to change gears smoothly. Yet given enough experience, if the instructor could distract you long enough for your subconscious to take over, you would carry out the gear changes without even knowing you were doing so. In light of this, it is worth contemplating the degree to which your subconscious does the driving for you the next time you cannot remember large portions of your journey, so engrossed were you in other matters.

By trying to move a new habit from the conscious mind to subconscious autonomy, you also confront an additional problem. In spite of not serving you well, the existing habit is inside your comfort zone, and the new way normally feels alien and uncomfortable. Your subconscious wants to reject it, since it does not want to move out of the comfort zone. For example, when trying to correct poor technique on your tennis backhand, the new method will tax your muscles in a different way. A better way, but something that initially feels alien. Despite being a well established correct technique, the new way will initially feel awkward, and your mind will urge you to resist and revert back to the comfort of your existing 'dodgy', but ever so familiar, sliced backhand.

And here comes another problem with our natural resistance to change – when we perform badly using the new method, we rapidly reject it as unworthy of further effort. We must remain diligent, repeating the new method, overriding the instinct to reject it. If we apply it often enough, it will bed in, and bear the fruits of its correctness. The subconscious will eventually start rejecting the old habit in favour of the new way when it can see tangible benefits. But until then, you must be stubborn in order to avoid regression. Also, if you do regress, there is a common inclination to treat such a regression as a sign of failure. But you must see it as merely a temporary setback, and get back on track in order to eventually succeed.

There is another pitfall to be wary of. If we start making progress with the new habit, we may plateau, and then fail to sense any progress at all. This may dishearten us and cause us to lose interest. We may actually not even see that we have made any progress at all. If we perform the same this week as last, we simply forget that the week before that we were less effective. Our memory can play tricks on us and jeopardise our efforts.

The concepts here are very pertinent to the rest of the book. If you are anything like me, many of your innate and acquired habits really do not serve you well, so you would need to work with the points raised above in order to successfully change. Just as the changing of a physical matter such as a tennis stroke will initially make you feel awkward, changing a mental behaviour will also make you feel awkward. During the transition from a bad mental habit to a better one, you will operate in a way that feels alien. You will literally not 'be yourself'. This simple matter alone creates a large failure rate in the adoption of new ways of approaching life. I laugh a lot more than I used to, often at things that are, in hindsight, actually not so funny. And it often does *feel* a bit contrived. But first of all, it does not matter if laughter is contrived – any form of laughter is beneficial. But the feeling I have is more that I would not normally have laughed rather than that the laugh is fabricated. I now realise that I simply find more things funny – adopting some of the ideas in the latter part of the book has had this delightful, and unexpected side effect.

But even such an overtly positive experience of laughing when you would have not have done so in the past can trigger a reversion back to past non-laughing habits because we may feel that we are not being true to ourselves. Personally, being true to myself simply with regard laughter does not serve me well – it is much better for me to be able to laugh more. So I change in order that laughing *becomes* my true self. But in the transition period, diligence and determination is required.

Note that the Alexander technique that resulted from his work is profound in its impact. Whilst it has subsequently been vindicated by research, many decades after its discovery, its very name labels it as "alternative health" rather than a matter of prime health. It is in fact a fundamental technique that needs a much higher status. Whilst the product of his detailed observations was a set of guidelines for improving posture, he also made it clear quite how much our habits stay entrenched. As I elucidated earlier, even habits that serve us poorly take an iron grip on us, stubbornly rejecting any replacement until it shows unequivocal advantages over the existing habit.

By habit here, I am of course moving beyond matters of posture, to matters of attitudes also. Genetically predicated habits are also not beyond the scope of change. Try to remember repeatedly that the human brain is a highly adaptive device. It grows, shrinks, and evolves in response to your life experiences, and your attitude towards them. Your genes in effect give it a starting path, but genes can be switched on and off by mere thought alone, allowing you much greater control over your destiny than you might imagine. In his interesting book "How your mind can heal your body", David Hamilton explores the extent of mind-body influence in great detail, along with the influence of your mind on your genetic expression. ^{HM}

For those who have read many self-help books, two matters about them should be fairly familiar. First, that the mere act of reading a self help book is itself very beneficial to health, in large part due to the general upbeat nature of its messages and anecdotes. Second, that this effect fades fairly quickly after finishing each book. The messages are rarely reinforced, and old habits swiftly reinstate themselves.

This is a huge shame, but it is avoidable with determination and persistence. You have to want to change, and have to persist with the change. And much as with the pursuance of a dream, you have to expect setbacks and not concede to them. When trying to change habits of *attitude*, this appears to be a hard nut to crack, but I have to repeat that the benefits are immense, much greater than you might imagine. One meta-benefit is that any one successful change can make your mind much receptive to subsequent changes.

When we start to adopt a new habit, Alexander discovered that we must not fight the old one. As Susan Jeffers says in "Feel the fear and do it anyway" [FF] :

"What we resist persists"

One of the ways in which old habits grip is us that they lie within our comfort zone, as mentioned before. Even a poorly executed tennis stroke, one that is less comfortable for the body, is comfortable to our mind by its very familiarity. That its awkwardness will eventually tire us prematurely is not recognised by the subconscious.

There is an additional benefit to be gained from moving outside of our comfort zones. They affect many areas of our lives, such as an avoidance of certain foreign foods, and even to the need to take the same route to work each day. By embracing new ways of living your life – by moving out of our comfort zones – we actually extend them. Sometimes, that can backfire, but often we grow as a result.

By way of example, one of my favourite hobbies is to talk with strangers. The more I can do so without discriminating, the more I accept people from all walks of life for what they are, and the more I start to see life from their perspectives. There is an undeniable risk in this exercise, for I may easily overstep the mark. Certainly, some cultures have very demanding social etiquette rules, and my occasional tendency to act tactlessly can readily expose me to the occasional social faux pas. But in general, the more I try to open myself up to others, the more I able to do it, and the more the new habit draws me in. I have never been very shy, but now I am more sociably capable through exercising this social skill, expanding beyond my comfort zone to include more and more people into my life.

The overriding method here is the intellect – your conscious intent to change. This capability was probably active in your youth, where you would choose to revise for exams at school, overriding the instinct to play instead. The long term goal is enforced by the intellect to override the fickleness of our emotions. Joe Dispenza devoted 500 pages to this concept in his excellent, but overly long book "Evolve your brain". [EB] I'll try in my own small way to pick out some key points he makes, and hope that I do justice to his concepts.

Joe explains that we start out in life with a largely blank slate, and are like sponges, soaking up experiences, and learning how to live life. We are necessarily highly influenced by family, friends and educational systems, and often blunder our ways through many situations. The net effect is that for the majority of us, many of the habits that we lay down in the pathways of the brain to help us cope are often not very effective, and sometimes counter effective. If our parents repeatedly told us we were useless, we would likely develop coping mechanisms that would essentially scar us for years or decades ahead.

The neocortex tends to handle new behaviours. As we develop and learn, these learned behaviours are gradually moved out of the neocortex to the subconscious parts of the brain where they can be handled automatically. Just picture how you learnt to ride a bicycle – you now do so without conscious thought. This is partly because the conscious mind is focused on dealing with novelty, but also because it is slow and lumbering, and the subconscious fast and efficient.

But the subconscious is also unquestioning. And this is the crux of a lot of our problems. We bury into our subconscious habits that do not serve us well because the subconscious does what it is told, and habits can get buried so deep that we are no longer aware of them, nor of their negative influence on our lives. Many such habits are behavioural responses to emotional situations – if your parents repeatedly told you that you would never amount to anything, you would be likley to underperform, and build habits that confirmed your parental labels, often unknowingly.

As we move from our twenties into our thirties, we move from a learning mindset into a 'doing' mindset. We can switch the autopilot on in an increasing number of situations, and this suits the body's need for economy of resources. If we had to consciously think about gear changes as we did when learning to drive, we would be exhausted each day simply driving to work. This is true for many interactions in our daily lives. The more that can be passed to the subconscious the better. When we are on subconscious autopilot, we are running efficiently, economically. We are in a comfort zone. And we get to like that feeling. So much so that it draws us in more and more as we age. Rather than live in awe and with openness to life as youngsters, we live more on autopilot, and effectively become less conscious. When on autopilot, we are only partially conscious. We tend to live along a stream of autopilot driven responses to life and the world around us.

Each time we reuse a tried and tested (but not necessarily beneficial) habit on autopilot, we reinforce the associated neural networks. The path becomes a rut, and we can struggle immensely to move away from it. If we try to consciously step along a new path, the brain will often resist, complaining that it prefers the tried and tested path, thank you very much. The brain and body can go so far onto the defensive that we start to release adrenaline and cortisone. And this uneasy, agitated state can get associated with the attempt to change our habits, and we often withdraw back to our comfort zone.

We can thus readily become victims of our own efficiencies, hugely coerced to stay within our comfort zones, even when they do us or the people around us no good. The vital point here is that we end up living according to how the environment feels to us, and to how we feel internally. We live in a kind of unconscious fog from hour to hour, and from day to day. To change the habits that serve us badly, we need to live more in our conscious mind. Only the wilful, determined and highly disciplined desire to change can effect that change. We have to gradually beat out a new neural path to encode a new habit, leaving the comfort of the well trodden path. We will frequently step back into the old rut, but discipline and will can move us back along the new route.

By repeatedly adhering to the new route, for example, by reasoning against the need for anger and thereby diffusing it rather than succumbing to it, the new way of being becomes established as a habit, and the old way dies off. The brain operates much like the muscles – use it or lose it. By no longer using the old anger habit, it fades in potency, replaced by the new calm response. And eventually, the new way becomes so habitual, the diligence required to establish and sustain it is no longer needed. We have literally changed our brain.

Before I finish here, it is worth pointing out that the new neural networks we have created in support of our new habit also act as attractants to other, positive and supportive ways of being. And the world will respond more positively to us as well, which will serve to reinforce your new personality even more. Very much a win-win situation.

That habits, and hence the brain, can be changed are also delightfully documented in "The brain that changes itself". A lady with severe balance difficulties was given an electronic device that fitted onto her tongue, sending electrical impulses in response to the spatial position of her limbs. Not only did her brain learn to use these signals in place of her body's missing proprioception signals, but the improved balance persisted for a few minutes *after* the device was removed. After many repeated trials, the effect of the device was extended to weeks and months following removal. [BR]

One of the ways, and indeed possibly the principle way in which the unfortunately named condition dyslexia arises is as a result of infant hearing difficulties, rather than shortcomings of intellect or effort. It appears that the auditory cortex fails to differentiate between closely spaced sounds, and thereby fails to recognise both the individual sounds, and, more crucially, their sequencing. This problem manifests in word learning and related difficulties. The 'Fast Forward' program [BR] sought to retrain these dyslexics by sounding words with large gaps between the phonemes (sound parts), so that they could identify the words, and then to gradually shorten these gaps. The effect was to retrain the brains of dyslexics, and their results were nothing short of spectacular.

Obsessive compulsive disorder (OCD) due to anxiety can equally be arrested by training. The method that appears to be most effective is to acquire an almost meditative, non judgemental observation of the compulsive urges to repeat behaviour, *without* conceding to these urges. Such impartial observations should be extended through to an observation of the *reaction* of your mind and body to not following the urge, again in a non-judgemental way. [PM] It takes great effort and time to calm down the OCD impulses, but it appears that a permanent change can be made to the OCD influence on your life. The brain demonstrates again its neuroplasticity.

I offer one final thought on habits before I turn towards the attitude you have towards yourself. A really neat way of stopping the negative trains of thoughts that can blight most of us is to carry around a click counter for a week or so, clicking at each instance of a negative thought. Initially, the click rate would be high, but the mere act of counting gives attention to these negative thoughts, and an innate desire to curb them develops. The daily counts normally reduce significantly within a week, leaving the clicker much happier as a result. This may appear to be a rare example of a focus on negativity that has a positive consequence, but in fact, the focus actually is on the *reduction* of clicks, rather than on the negative thoughts themselves.

Chapter Nineteen
Attitude to self

I have shown you earlier that happiness is essentially a by product of our attitude to life. However, happiness is also affected by the attitude we have to ourselves. We should cultivate respect for ourselves – we should develop a high self-esteem. Alas, our self-esteem can be heavily assaulted in modern times, not least as a result of the exploitation of our emotions by capitalism. Marketing departments play on vulnerabilities in our self-esteem as a means of selling more products. We are made to feel inadequate if we fall short both on material possessions, and in our appearance. Society also imposes many demands on us to conform, threatening to treat us as inferior if we do not. In summary, it is all too easy to suffer damage to our self-esteem as a result of external influences.

In addition to external assaults, we are also affected internally, where a stream of subconscious chatter continually informs us of its appraisal of our ongoing performance in the game of life. (The 'chatterbox' I described when I discussed meditation). Eugene Sagan describes the subconscious as a 'pathological critic' when engaged in this form of chatter. [SE] This 'critic' punishes us for the mistakes we make, and taunts us for being perceived as inferior to others. It often emphasises the negative and de-emphasises the positive. And because we are so easily fooled into believing that these criticisms were created by our conscious thought, we tend to accept them without question. Why question your own mind? This has the twin effect of lowering our self-esteem and of reinforcing the validity and power of these subconscious thoughts.

It has been observed, however, that optimists tend to have a more supportive subconscious, and hence a healthier self-esteem and life. That they are oblivious to some of their shortcomings is more a problem for others than for themselves. It would appear that psychopaths have the best deal with regard subconscious criticism. And in this regard, they are polar opposites of the sensitive, worrying type of person.

Making mistakes is a fundamental part of the human condition – we have actually even evolved to make mistakes. If you try to avoid making mistakes, you are essentially avoiding life. Conversely, by embracing life and taking risks, you live a richer life, but thereby expose yourself to more mistakes. By allowing yourself to make mistakes, and avoid punishing yourself using hindsight, you can relax and also become more spontaneous. I personally often become silly when I relax. I suspect that this happens as a release valve for too much time caught up in the seriousness of tension headaches. But I learn now not to apologise too often for my silliness. I mean to do no harm, and by letting my hair down, I am more likely to be more relaxed, fun company. By freeing yourself from hindsight-driven responsibility for mistakes, your health and self-esteem can be enhanced.

A low self-esteem can also result from poor parenting, where children are often belittled or given inconsistent and conflicting guidance. All children misbehave, and a good parent will reprimand the child for the behaviour. A bad parent will label the child as bad, rather than the behaviour – each individual misdemeanour is scaled up to a generalised level. Repeated often enough, such generalised chastisements will cause the afflicted children to start to label themselves as bad, unable to differentiate between them-self and their behaviours. This poor parenting is actually a form of child cruelty.

Childhood labels and self-limiting behaviours are often carried through to adulthood out of sight of conscious awareness. They get internalised and their power over us gets forgotten (see the last chapter). As adults, we can subsequently fail to recognise the influence of these internalised forces. They become ingrained in us as children, and become automatic behaviours, relegated to the subconscious. And some become core-beliefs, affecting a wide range of issues and generally steering us in wrong directions.

For example, if a parent were to instill in a child that they should always do what someone tells them to do, then they are priming the child for many problems of subservience later in life. This is bad parenting, and if such a 'should' is repeated enough, as is often the case, it becomes a mandate – a hardened core-belief for the poor child. The future tendency of such a child to please others would be very hard to shake off, yet they would be unlikely to relate their subservient behaviour back to their childhood priming. Each time they let someone down, they would punish themselves because their parents had essentially programmed them, through repetition, to believe that this was absolutely bad to let anyone down for any reason. I recommend "The disease to please" by Harriet Braiker if this particular plight affects you. [DP]

The tendency to have 'shoulds' and 'musts' in our repertoire is widespread. They are generally indicative of misguided value systems. We can reverse them by simply challenging them, and doing so often enough breaks the habit. But I emphasise again that it takes resolution and persistence, and of course a robust desire to change, along with a belief that change is possible. I do not apologise for endlessly repeating this advice, since failure to follow through personal change is all too common.

I'll give you an example of a 'should'. When I play tennis against a a much weaker player and lose, my instinct is to feel anger and disgust that this should happen. These emotions appear swiftly, before I can think, driven in my case by a core belief that stronger players 'should' not be beaten by weaker players. It is best not to fight the feelings, but to challenge that core belief. First, I say to myself that the defeat has happened and cannot be reversed. There is literally no use in crying over spilt milk. Second, it may be that I deserved to lose because I played poorly, or that he played the game of his life, or some combination of these two. Your core beliefs are often too simplistic to take such matters into account, and often act bluntly on their basic premise. Third, I try to see the 'problem' of losing as an opportunity to learn. To find out where

I went wrong. By focusing forwards rather than backwards, I diffuse the anger and can develop instead.

If you succumb to the pathological critic that blames you for losing to a weaker player, you merely serve to strengthen that critic. You are accepting its punishment and expressing it in the form of anger. By rationalising the defeat instead, you replace punishment with action, and weaken the critic. [SE]

Chronic low self-esteem results when we see each failure we make as defining us. This has been an ongoing problem with myself and also of one of my sisters. As a professional photographer, each wedding I photographed would invariably bring moments of difficulty, and any consequent shortcoming in my performance would stand out in my memories ahead of any good work I had done. Not only would each wedding shoot be largely defined by my failings, I would also label myself as an inadequate photographer by virtue of this distorted focus. This focus would often blind me to all the good things I would do on the day.

I have every reason to believe that my sister, Carol, is not only a capable and effective secondary school Mathematics teacher, but a much loved one. However, she can often fall into the trap of labelling herself as a poor teacher by virtue of a single bad lesson. I remember once she told me about a Friday night 'I have not been sacked' celebration meal she had with her family. It transpires that someone had sat in her classroom, apparently monitoring her performance at a time when she had been experiencing some minor difficulties. Because no one had told her about this person, she had assumed the worst – that she was being appraised for possible bad performance. The head master duly apologised for failing to inform her of the role of this person, and to clarify that she was in no way a bad teacher. He declared that he would be devastated if he lost her as a teacher from his school.

There are two big aids to self-esteem that we really all should be taught in school. The first is to love ourselves. And yes, it is easy to see why this is rarely taught. In many countries, it is a social taboo to actually have warm and compassionate feelings towards oneself, as if such needs should only be proffered to others. Respecting, loving, and caring for yourself is not as narcissistic as it sounds. By treating yourself in a loving, supportive way, you give yourself time out to rest when needed, and are then of course better able to help others. It is no good wearing yourself out in the service of others to the point where you are no good to anyone. Help yourself in order to be able to help others – get the balance right and everyone gains.

Second, that we are rarely told that we are not actually personally responsible for our genetic inheritance. I did not choose to have a slightly nervous disposition. I did not choose to have a long neck and balding hair. I did not choose to have a pedantic nature. Do not take blame for these things – do not *punish* yourself for your genetic shortcomings. You can, and should, however, take *responsibility* for working around them.

By way of example, I have inherited a family trait of occasional tendency to irritability. I accept this plight, and do my best to reason away the feelings when they occur, and avoid situations that might trigger them. The fact that I get irritable in the first place is not really my fault. It is something that happens *to me* more than *by me*. I give myself some *slack*, and also some *credit* for my efforts in compensating for and reconciling genetically sourced difficulties. It is important that you too give yourself time to learn how to handle inherited difficulties. As Paul Gilbert puts it so eloquently in "The Compassionate Mind" CM :

"I find it amazing that so many of the desires that flow through me, and indeed all of us, were designed not only before me but before all humans."

A key here is to let your self-esteem be guided by a holistic picture of who you are. You should see your weaknesses in balance with your strengths. And it is best to see each 'failure' as an individual event. You are not the behaviour – you are the person performing the behaviour. Let your self-esteem be guided by the whole picture and not individual events. As a very simple, but surprisingly common example, stop calling yourself a failure each time you make a mistake. This tendency to lose self-esteem can also strangely apply to positive events. When you achieve something good, your self-esteem receives a boost, but if you invest too much weight in such highs, then your self-esteem is equally fragile. See achievements as the icing on the cake, and move on. Likewise, rather than be dragged down by mistakes, learn from them, and also move on. It is also crucial that you let your self-esteem be independent of the opinions of others. We can fall into the danger of being controlled by their opinions, leaving ourselves open to even the tiniest slight.

As an aside now, I am intentionally being honest and forthright in this book about my own shortcomings. A lot of them are a consequence of the highly sensitive and emotional predisposition that my genes have given to me. Now, aged 53, I am able to realise that I have always been much less the instigator of many of my shortcomings, and much more a witness or victim of them. As a consequence, I can happily discuss them without any impact on my self-esteem. If there appear to be a lot of shortcomings, then so be it – I drew a genetic short straw – and deserve credit for handling them. You may have genetically based shortcomings that you are not happy with. I do not want to make you aware of them now in a negative sense. I want you to accept them as and when this book makes you aware of them and improve your health as a consequence. There is a whole chapter on this matter of acceptance coming up.

Criticism and confrontation are two of my achilles heels. I have tended to take all forms of criticism to heart, adopting an emotionally defensive, but submissive stance. Much like with anger, if I pause, and do not engage immediately with my instinctively rapid emotional reaction to criticism, then I can handle it more rationally. Frequently, I find, the criticism is ill founded, and often just an outburst from someone who is using the criticism to deflect away from their own ill feelings. But if the criticism is indeed justified, it is much better to take action rather than dwell on feelings of hurt. Try to rectify the cause of the criticism rather than become submerged in reactive emotions. Again, treat the criticism as an individual event, and do not see as a defining you or your self-esteem.

On the soccer field recently, I noticed that a friend of mine is all too apt to criticise my posture when we practice passing the ball. His tone is very denigrating, and until recently, I took offence. But now I look for the message and not the voice, and see if he has a point to make. Often, however, he is simply being harsh, failing to realise that we are not all as naturally gifted as he is. His agenda appears to be one of self inflation at my expense. I recognise this and can laugh at his verbal attacks. I do try to improve, but I generally do not let his criticism get to me.

If criticism is vague or unreasonable, ask the criticising person in a calm tone for clarification. Your tone should immediately start to calm the critic, as they are often looking for a negative reaction rather than to help you. If they remain vague, but you keep asking for clarification, they are less likely to verbally attack you in this way in the future. If you bite, and react to the vague criticism, then they will be more likely attack you again in the future. The ultimate diffuser of criticism is calm agreement. "Yes, you are right, I do talk a lot. I am, however, simply being friendly, and do try to recognise when I over do it, but cannot always get the balance right." What can they then say?

Turning to confrontation, I refer to the ability to both handle it when it naturally arises from criticism, for example, but also to be able to actively and comfortably use confrontation with someone who is being unreasonable to you. It may be as simple as telling the waiter that your food is cold. Or to confront someone who is stepping over the mark.

I personally have a big problem with confronting people in a calm way. I strongly believe that this problem arises from my childhood, where I *always* acceded to my father's demands because of the threat of his raised voice. He was, it appears, happy to use strong emotional force to get what he wanted. And it was much easier to be submissive in order to keep the peace than it was to to confront him. As a consequence of failing to confront him and live with his emotional threats until he backed down, I now have so strong a rise in emotions when I even *think* about confrontation that I tend to avoid even starting.

The best way to handle confrontation is to do so calmly without an engagement of emotions. This is hard for me because of such rapid emotional inflammation in anticipation of a negative outcome of such confrontation. My father essentially, and unwittingly, trained me to expect an emotional onslaught every time I tried to face up to someone. But I will work on this, and hope to be able to face the world better as a consequence of addressing this problem. I will be healthier as a result of being able to take a reasonable stand, and will be able to do so more easily the more often I succeed.

If you believe that your childhood programming is working against you, as it evidently is for me, then the mind and behaviour improving technique called Cognitive Behaviour Therapy (CBT) that I cover in the next chapter can help enormously. You may also benefit from a visit to a friendly psychotherapist. You might, however, dismiss such an idea as a form of defeat – an admission that you are mentally ill. Sadly, mental illness is heavily stigmatised, but it really, really should not be. A greater proportion of the population probably have some form of mental illness than physical illness. Depression, for example, is extremely common. It is so much healthier to see mental illness as a lack of mental health. A slightly depressed mood may be deemed equivalent to a mild cold, for example. Besides, it shows a strength of character to arrange for psychotherapy – to take action on your condition. The whole point about psychotherapy, whether administered by yourself or by a therapist, is that it can tease out bad habits, behaviours and core-beliefs (schemas) and release you from their grip.

It might help if I relate my own personal experience of psychotherapy treatment. I visited Heather in the Winter of 2009 with the hope of releasing trapped emotions that I felt might be the cause of my chronic tension headaches. Whilst we did address these headaches and their possible causes, and I duly cried away a lot of feelings held from my childhood, it did not seem to help them. At least not at that time.

But Heather is a very agile therapist, and was able to unearth many habits in my thinking that were letting me down, not least that I was not giving myself anywhere near enough credit for the many skills and abilities I have. It is, sadly, a social habit of the British to play down skills and achievements of ourselves and of others. But a British therapist does not have to stick to such a convention, and was able to reflect back to me the reality of the gifts I have. The penny eventually dropped – my self-esteem was appropriately enriched by a true awareness of the gifts that I bring to the world. Esteem enhanced by value. But a value that I previously dismissed because I felt that it was inherited rather than earned. For the world which receive the cabinets and drawings I can produce, or the photographs I take, it matters not what proportion of their production was from gift or from effort.

Another aspect of self esteem that she explored was my instinctive tendency to apologise. To basically apologise for being who I am! This was of course a large and easy matter to start to address. When it slowly dawned on me that neither I nor the world gained from such an attitude, I decided to stop apologising for who I am and what I do. Two days later, I went to the pub to watch a soccer match before trying to mimic the football skills I saw in a game with my friends in the park. As I sat with a group of youngsters in that pub, I started easing myself into their conversation. After a while, however, I noticed that they often failed to respond to what I said. Eventually, they presumably got used to my voice and deemed what I had to say to be relatively interesting, so responded better.

Up until then, I would normally have reacted poorly to being ignored. I would have sensed that what I had to say was not interesting enough, or poorly timed, so I would work harder and harder to grab their attention, or just go quiet, blaming myself in both instances. But this time, I was aware of my normal apologetic response to the situation. I was also aware that I was making only few comments, and so realised that these youngsters were actually at fault – they were blanking me out without actually knowing me. They were being rude to me, and my low self-esteem in the past had blinded me to that sort of thing.

Gosh, how relaxed I then felt!. It was a huge weight lifted from my shoulders. My low self esteem had so often pointed the finger of guilt at myself in any situation of social failure, regardless of who was truly the culprit. By removing this core sense of apology about myself, I not only relaxed where before I would tense, but I was able to see the world without the taint of low-self-esteem bias – these boys were simply being rude and ignorant.

Delightfully, there was more enlightenment to follow at the park, as my now reinforced anti-apologetic attitude was given a new situation to deal with. My football abilities are genuinely relatively limited in comparison to many of my friends, and I used to apologise frequently for each and every mistake I made. This day, I decided to reduce this to a bare minimum. And a number of interesting things transpired as a result.

First, I noticed how many other players were making mistakes. Indeed, no player was exempt from making mistakes. My previous focus on my own shortcomings had literally blinded me to this reality.

Second, that there were others who also occasionally apologised for their mistakes. I had rarely noticed this before.

Third, that the best player not only made mistakes, but used a psychological device to blind others and himself to his shortcomings. He would either blame those around him for failing to forewarn him of a player tackling the ball away from his feet, or he would blame the pitch. The realisation that he and others were using this deflection mechanism had eluded me for years. These players are so much more concerned about retaining a high sense of self that they transfer their shortcomings elsewhere. I was previously blinded by his use of psychology to sustain a high playing status with himself and others. And I actually suspect that he is himself probably unaware that he does this.

Fourth, my liberation from apology meant that I could relax, and focus on playing rather than on any possible failures in my play. I actually had not guessed this relaxation would happen, nor what was to follow. The consequences of a restored self-esteem was spreading further than I had expected. In the past, when the ball was passed to me, I would swiftly seek to distribute it to someone else, in fear of being dispossessed. A reflection of low self opinion. Now, I found myself pausing, and even nutmegging players who approached me (nutmeg is a British expression, meaning to play the ball through a player's legs). Or I would feint one way and then skip the other way past another player.

This release from apology had reawakened the abilities that I was in a sense apologising for not having. You have no idea how sweet this was. My apologetic attitude had made me absorb all criticisms of my play in the past, and to deflect all compliments as being one-offs. And now it was almost a reverse situation. Note that there is a parallel here with the negative stance that governmental advisers adopt, allowing the momentum of faulty past decisions to blind themselves to the reality of research that contradicted them.

In the space of just two days, I had mostly lifted the effect this apologetic attitude was having on my self esteem. And this after decades where I had inculcated this self-demeaning habit. Almost as surprisingly, I have pretty much kept the urge to apologise at bay. Some psychotherapy can indeed be this remarkably fast and effective, out of all proportion to the period of original suffering.

Chapter Twenty
The wrong kind of thinking

Much as you are what you eat, you are also very much what you think. Indeed, what you think has a much greater bearing on your health than you might imagine. The wrong kind of thinking can set you up for many health problems. David Burns was one of the founders of Cognitive Behaviour Therapy (CBT), a set of techniques that look to correct such damaging patterns of thinking. His comprehensive book on the subject "Feeling Good" maybe goes too far in its premise that 'All moods are determined by thought', but it is still a very valuable resource for helping with the wrong kind of thinking. [FG] I'll cover the key concepts here, and put my own spin on them, but recommend that book for more in-depth reading.

In a sense, CBT is a loose variation of the Alexander technique. Habits of mind, including those that do not serve you well, are akin to habits of posture, or of sporting technique. We are largely unaware of how much they affect our health, and have to again use due diligence and patience to realign them to help rather than hinder our lives. The results of such diligence are likely to be well worth the effort.

From my perspective, I believe that strong emotions can readily establish and perpetuate the wrong kinds of thinking. Remember that emotions can engage before reason has time to get started (the principal emotional centre of the brain, the amygdala, is the target for many sensory inputs, which it vets before the conscious mind responds). If our emotions are strong enough, they can start blinkering and distorting our

171

thinking. When gripped by anger, for example, the brain shifts into a state where it will focus on information that supports the anger agenda, and is literally incapable of handling positive thoughts, or anti-anger concepts. Evolution has given us, in anger, a highly focused and efficient mechanism for swift attainment of a goal – the correction of a perceived injustice. But strong emotions like anger do not fit well into modern life, and can disturb the balance in our thinking, setting us up for long term bad thinking patterns. Whilst this is my conjecture, it does seem to be born out by experience.

Before I go on to describe the details of CBT, it is worth noting that research has not only shown it to be largely as effective as drugs such as anti-depressants, but also that the areas of the brain affected by CBT tend to ensure a longer term retention of the benefits. It calms down the frontal cortex, for example, and strengthens the hippocampus – that region responsible for engaging with the world that is also strengthened by exercise. [PM] In light of what I have told you earlier about anti-depressants, it seems that our placebo handling of depression (in the guise of an anti-depressant tablet) is not quite so effective as revamping our thinking. It is likely that the placebo effect is an anaesthetising one, and the revamping a redirecting one, and hence likely to have longer term benefits.

Whilst a fair proportion of the world's population can be described as optimistic, in general, humans are genetically programmed to readily adopt a negative, defensive stance. Over millions of years, pessimistic thinking has generally been vital for survival purposes (those that took a risk too far did not survive to live another day). Much negative thinking, however, involves many inaccurate judgements and projections into the future. [FG] But this genetic heritage need not be a mandate. CBT can realign even genetic tendencies because the human brain is very happy to flex and adapt.

The standard 10 CBT thinking failings are shown on the following page. For each I give one or two illustrative examples.

1   **All or nothing thinking.**
"I only got grade B – I am useless."
After a failed date : "I'll never get a girlfriend."

2   **Over generalisation.**
"All women are the same."

3   **Mental filtering.**
Focusing on a bad answer to one question in an exam, and forgetting that you did a brilliant job on all the other questions.

4   **Disqualifying the positive.**
"Sure I got a hole in one, but what about that double bogey?"

5   **Jumping to conclusions.**
This comes in two flavours.
Mind reader: "Did you see the look she gave me? She cannot possibly like me."
Fortune teller : "If I see her too soon after the last date she might get bored with me."

6   **Magnifying and minimising.**
In essence this is a variation on 3 and 4.
Magnification : A single mistake takes on huge proportions
Minimisation : You help a friend out but then dismiss this as something anyone would do.

7   **Emotional reasoning.**
"I feel so guilty that I must be guilty."

8   **Shoulds and musts.**
"I should be nice to everyone."
"I must turn up or they will hate me."

9   **Labelling and mislabelling.**
"I missed the easiest of shots. I must be rubbish."

10   **Personalisation.**
When a mother sees a bad school report card, she thinks she must be a bad parent.

Whilst the examples of the wrong kinds of thinking may be obvious, it is probably worth labouring each point, to drive home the 10 CBT messages :

1. All or nothing thinking

The impulsive response that exam grade B is an indicator of universal failure is of course an overreaction to the expected A grade. By holding onto the whole picture of your self esteem at all times, you can let the emotion ride and see this slight shortcoming in a better light. One mistake does not define you. Nor does the result in one exam trap you on a path of failure – there are far too many millionaires who failed miserably at school for that to be the case. Likewise, the failed date means only that tonight was not so good. You cannot predict the future from it. But if you do believe you can, the failure is more likely to become a core-belief, and a self-fulfilling belief at that.

2. Over generalisation

Intellectually, you do know that women are different. The flippancy of the statement is again emotionally driven because yet another woman has failed to live up to your expectations. You are taking the lazy route, and not using your intelligence.

3. Mental filtering

By obsessing on one poor answer in an exam, you are failing to see the forest for the trees. You are allowing the emotional weight attached to this single failure to blight the whole exam. Detaching from the emotional overreaction will give you a more balanced perspective.

4. Disqualifying the positive

A hole in one should be an excuse for celebration. Forget the rest of the card – enjoy this rarest of golfing achievements!

5. Jumping to conclusions

A friend of mine struggled to hold onto relationships because he put too much weight on every detail. It really only did take one unexpected look from his new date to see him disappear in a cloud of dust. At the very least, he should have gently spoken to her and asked her how she was, rather then guess. In all likelihood, her expression was fleeting and a reflection of other matters on her mind. By being fixated on the opinions of others, my poor friend was leaving himself open to problems such as this. With the other issue, seeing a girl too soon after the first date can indeed be a problem. But all you have to do, and all you really can do, is to make a decision. Take the risk of seeing her soon, if this is your heart's desire, or bide your time. Predicting her response will get you nowhere since only time will reveal that.

6. Magnifying and minimising

The mistake taking on huge proportions is akin to the grade B in the exam when A was expected. Helping a friend is a good deed. Don't go overboard in self praise, but do give yourself credit – you are then more likely to do it again in the future.

7. Emotional reasoning

Reality and your emotional assessment are often misaligned. Find out the truth about the guilty party rather than jumping to self blame. If you are to blame, do not dwell on the matter, but seek to make amends.

8. Shoulds and musts

Tempering the grip that the 'should' and 'must' core beliefs hold on you is key here. From an intellectual standpoint, it makes no sense to have inflexible rules like these. If you are extremely tired and a friend wants you to go out to a party, thinking that you should go is unwise – you will only likely sit there and struggle to mix in.

9. Labelling and mislabelling

You are not defined by your actions or emotions. Missing an easy shot does not change who you are, as long as you do not let it. Again, keeping a holistic view of yourself is crucial. In the context of your whole life, the odd mistake is perfectly acceptable. Even if frustrating.

10. Personalisation

There may be many reasons for a poor report card. Impulsively jumping to conclusions stops you enquiring into the real picture. It may be that your child is being bullied and cannot concentrate. Fixing this problem will help your child, your relationship with your child and probably the rest of the class also.

Whilst there is merit in these designations, and they have of course served the CBT practitioners well for many years, they seemed to be an untidy, overlapping set of faulty thinking categories. So I have attempted to normalise them in order that the basis of faulty thinking be more clearly understood. I also added a new category that is a particular problem for me :

A   Amplifying negativity
- Blowing a negative event out of proportion.
- Generalising negativity as a constant.
- Allowing the negative to blind you to the positive.

B   Extrapolating from few clues
- Guessing what has happened, is happening, or will happen.

C   Assuming too much responsibility
- Putting extreme demands on yourself.
- Assuming that you are more likely than others to be at fault.
- Assuming that you are the one who needs to act first when others don't.

D   Trying to control too much
- Having too many expectations about how things should be.
- Getting too affected when expectations are not met.

As I said, category D is a major problem for me, try as I might to counter it. I suspect that being on the autistic spectrum is a factor, making me overly affected by changes of routine. It might amuse you to know that I ticked all 10 CBT boxes, although I suspect that many others would do so also.

The key mechanism that CBT uses to address such destructive thinking patterns is to record them on paper. Many CBT readers will likely skip this part of the process, believing that reading and applying the concepts in daily life is enough. But the point of keeping a diary of unsupportive mental behaviours is to focus more intently on them.

CBT is also involved in tackling the underlying core beliefs that often fuel erroneous thinking patterns. To trace back existing thinking problems to core beliefs is quite involved. "Feeling Good" provides templates and methods for doing this. [FG] The crucial factor in the success of such methods is in their due application. I repeat again that it is not sufficient to read a self help book – you must apply its methods. Without doing so, it does not matter if the methods look too simple to need paper work. You will achieve very little without following the due process. It is akin to reading a muscle building book without lifting a finger. For once, bureaucracy is important.

"The compassionate mind" by Paul Gilbert very elegantly explains how the brain is in effect split into 2 parts. [CM] The so-called old brain, present in humans for millions of years was principally involved in base functions that served to satisfy human needs for shelter, food, sex, defence and attack. Emotions such as anger played a pivotal role. The so-called new brain, especially the frontal cortex (a much more recent product of evolution), is involved in higher functions such as thinking, reasoning, exploring and socialising. We can choose to let the base functions rule, or let the higher functions steer a better direction. We can therefore lessen the damage of base functions where they have no meaningful place in modern life. CBT in a sense takes this approach, steering us away from emotionally charged thinking patterns.

A class of schoolchildren may be genetically predisposed to be unruly, succumbing to their emotions. Fun though this is for them, if it is left unaddressed, the children may grow into adults with social problems. Fuel your emotions too much and you fail to evolve your higher functions. In a sense, it is as if we have two competing minds – the old and new. If we fuel the new, rational mind, then we reinforce it and live a healthier life, and release the grip of the emotional old brain on our lives.

This is not to say that we should become emotionless. Or that we should never feel emotions such as anger again. It is more that we should not allow unsupportive emotions to *control* us. It is much better to encourage laughter for example, and reason away anger, jealousy and other such emotions. You are not defined by your emotions, so do not let them define you. They are transient, and just a reflection of your current state of play – you are separate from them. Do not be drawn into living life through them as they will come and go. [15]

As an aside, I want to relate my own experience of the emotion we call jealousy. When I listen to the radio whilst suffering a bad headache, I find that I am jealous of the upbeat tone of the presenters. I see their mood elevated above mine on many days. I do not try to fuel this jealousy as it does me no good.

And the futility of doing so was recently wonderfully brought home by a story about a certain Sir Paul McCartney, the ex-Beatle singer/song-writer. I have always maintained that he has lived a fabulously rich and enjoyable life, and yet is very grounded and humble in nature, taking life in his stride. I always used to cite his life as a prime example of a very lucky, fulfilled and happy one. But I was recently informed that he has laboured for decades with an inferiority complex towards John Lennon, to the point where he has recently been working hard to reverse the song author credits from 'Lennon and McCartney' to 'McCartney and Lennon'. In spite of a staggeringly rich life, even Paul McCartney can get embroiled in petty and self destructive jealousy!

Chapter Twenty One

Fear, anxiety and panic

Whilst faulty thinking can cause us many problems, as you have seen, it is my opinion that emotional problems can cause significantly greater damage to health. Emotions such as fear can not only paralyse you, but severely limit your involvement in life as you seek to avoid situations that can trigger that emotion. Fear can have the marginalisation effects that I covered earlier with injury and illness. It is often made worse by the social stigmatisation of sufferers, and cruel and unthinking though this is, it is a reality that has to be faced by many.

Fear is a form of habit. An emotionally triggered one that is self perpetuating. Fear is an emotion that grips so strongly that it feeds itself. It is deeply sad in my viewpoint that fear is an example of a nasty asymmetry in life. After decades happily stroking all shapes and sizes of dogs, I encountered a tiny, innocuous looking one a few years ago who decided to bite me, drawing blood. This event lasted just a few seconds, but it has taken years since to slowly remove the fear of a further dog bite that was kindled on that day. This ratio of a few seconds to a few years is highly asymmetric. The overly defensive nature of our minds can create such protracted problems. I try to stroke each dog I meet, and slowly I have eased away this fear that the next dog will bite. But it really has faded slowly. This is partly because my intelligence interferes – I do know that dogs can be unpredictable, and generally do care if they bite someone. They are animals after all. So my thinking can fuel the overt defensiveness my mind wants to adopt towards dogs since that bite. But, like all habits, fear can be tackled, even though it can sometimes take a long time.

As is obvious from the title of her popular little book "Face the fear and do it anyway", Susan Jeffers strongly believes that we must not live a life in avoidance of fear, but instead literally seek out that fear. [FF] This is somewhat more proactive than confronting fear when it appears. We are advised to literally seek out fear so that we may banish it. However, as I illustrated, we must not expect the act of facing the fear to *remove* the fear. You *will* feel fearful when you face it, and the key of course is to hang in there. You desensitise yourself to the fear by facing it. When you repeat the act the next time the fear will be less powerful. But there is an additional benefit to facing the fear. We strengthen our self respect – our self-esteem is bolstered. And this is not a temporary lift. Removal of a fear yields a long standing benefit. The very act of tackling a fear is also a boost to our self-esteem. Although it too is a one off event, it clues us into our potential to apply the same bravery to other fears and situations.

One of the softer manifestations of fear is that of making mistakes. As mentioned before, humans are virtually designed to make mistakes. To be human is to err. In most cases, you do not set out to make mistakes, so you are unwise to use hindsight to punish yourself. [RA] Not least also because the mistake is now history. Better to make amends for the mistake if necessary and learn from it.

A precursor to a fearful event can be a brooding anxiety. It is a kind of preemptive fear, such as experienced prior to an exam, where the anxiety is an expression of the fear of failing the exam. Given enough fearful situations and anxiety, it can become generalised – we can acquire an ever present background edginess, keeping us on general guard against what life is likely to throw our way. As you might expect, this generalised anxiety, or chronic anxiety, is much more prevalent in highly sensitive people.

According to Elaine Aron in her book "The Highly Sensitive Person"[HS], around 20% of the population are highly sensitive, and a matching 20% are highly insensitive. Neither trait is right or wrong – they each have pros and cons – although the highly **in**sensitive tend to cope better with life, and are generally socially more accepted. In the US, sensitive types are often seen as weak, and anti-social, especially if also shy. I probably cope well because whilst sensitive, I am far from shy, and can often defend my sensitivity with words. In a sense, the highly sensitive person is the polar opposite of the psychopath. Whilst sensitives are highly tuned into social conformance, often punishing themselves for social failings, psychopaths are liberated from social conformance, and can bludgeon their way through life with barely a care.

Being highly sensitivity allows even simple things to be perceived more intensely, with great pleasure readily achieved from innocuous activities such as reading quietly in the corner, away from the madding crowd. But this sensitivity also tends to *need* that kind of isolation – to avoid sensory overload. Whilst I really enjoy a good conversation, my sensitivity makes me aware of so many facets of what is spoken, of the undercurrents in the other people talking, that after an hour, I actually normally need to take a rest. A highly insensitive person, by contrast, could happily sit in company all day, as even the most engaging conversation is not terribly stimulating for them. They have the converse problem of urges to seek high thrill levels. A highly insensitive person might leave the bar with the group he was chatting with to go dancing, whilst the sensitive person slips away to go home and relax in font of the TV. And it is all too easy for the sensitive person to feel inferior because his tendency to overload can take him out of the mainstream of life. Their quiet way of life suits them, but they are looked down upon by the majority.

Just like the isolation with injuries and illness, isolation caused by sensory overload can marginalise you, with all that entails. So the harmful effects of isolation and generalised anxiety can blight the life of sensitive people. I am sensitive and almost aspergic, so I am personally very aware of these matters. And the key to my sanity, drawn from my own growth in self-esteem, is to recognise that I do not have to fit into any social stereotype. If one good chat a day in the coffee shop is enough social stimulation for me, then so be it. If I spend vast hours, as I do, in my own company, where interruptions and noise from others is removed, and that this suits me very much, then so be it also. I am not being anti-social at all – more that I am becoming more accepting of what makes me tick. My stress levels lower, I generally thoroughly enjoy my sojourns to the coffee shop, and the order in my life. And my anxiety levels stay at lower levels also. Routines and predictability are the mainstays of sanity and health for sensitive and autistic types. If sensitives can accept how they are built, rather than overload themselves by trying to be like insensitives, then they will live healthier lives.

Chronic anxiety and unexpressed emotions can express themselves in muscular tightness, especially in the back of the neck. [RA] And this is likely to be the cause of my tension headaches. Note that attempts to alleviate the muscular tension are likely to fail. The tension is symptomatic, and the underlying emotional causes need to be addressed instead. Hence my attempts to use a psychotherapist to unleash trapped emotions from my past. I suspect that I simply did not persist long enough with that line of enquiry. Or possibly that the muscle tension expression of trapped emotions has persisted so long that it has become a habit completely detached from the original cause.

A debilitating effect of chronic anxiety is that energy levels and stamina are often lowered. And this can mistakenly lead the sufferer to believe that they should avoid overwork. And certainly to avoid stressful situations. But the paradox is that *positive* stress can benefit the sufferer. Each day I spend writing, I get so embroiled in the process that I tend to forget my headaches. And research has shown that distraction from pain not only takes your focus away from it, but that the pain levels in the brain actually reduce when attention is moved away from them. [EB] What we attend to in the mind becomes our reality. By the end of each day, I generally find that I have been totally unaware of any headache. They may then have reappear when I stopped writing, but I have established a pattern now where I push myself to write as much as I can, often beyond the levels of tiredness where I would normally think it sensible to stop. This is very much the positive type of stress I am referring to. It is not a stress of conflict except in the very loose sense that I am working when my body it s asking for rest. But the point here is that my body is only asking to stay in a comfort zone. The more I can do each day, the more that I will comfortably be able to do in future days.

Chronic anxiety can draw you into its lair. If you focus on anxious feelings, and fall into the trap of reading the worst into them, you merely fuel them. Waves of anxiety can develop into extreme peaks that are called panic attacks. And you guessed right that I too have suffered with these. I can assure you that not even a hypochondriac would be likely enough to wish them upon himself. They are an intensely petrifying experience where you fear at the very least that a heart attack is imminent, and often that your time is up. I believe it a criminally poor choice of words to describe such events as 'panic attacks'. Such a loose, mild description of one of the most terrifying experiences you might suffer is grossly misleading to those who might seek to help the sufferer. It implies a brief and almost trivial loss of perspective. The reality is that the extreme state of anxiety that peaks in a panic attack releases so much adrenalin and cortisol that your heart-rate is raised to a very high level, you can become very light headed, can suffer severe breathing difficulties, can have a tight band across your chest and in general feel desperately ill. The intensity of panic attacks urges action, yet you neither know what to do, nor have the capacity to act anyway, so crippling are they. These panic attacks are an extreme form of the 'fight or flight' defence posture. Or rather, they are a third type of response to a perceived threat. We freeze. We claustrophobically freeze. We are paralysed by extreme fear.

If these panic attacks are alien to you, just be grateful. Be very grateful! Because there is a also a nasty corollary to them. Whilst it is your brain that is generating the attack, it is so intense that your brain then forges an association with your surroundings at the time of the attack, *even if the surroundings had nothing to do with the attack*. And similar surroundings in the future can then be a trigger for a repeat attack. The brain perversely works against itself – it gets so upset with the feelings of the current attack that it marks everything – including the environment – as causal. When you are slightly anxious in a similar environment in the future, a panic attack can spontaneously occur.

However, it is possible to calm panic attacks down, and eventually reduce their frequency and intensity. I am personally indebted for help on this matter to the small but brilliant "Self help for your nerves" by Clare Weeks. [SH] I gave a copy of this book to a friend who had started to suffer panic attacks after suffering a stroke whilst relatively young. It helped her enormously also.

As Weeks explains, any nervous disorder, such as panic attacks, and even a slide towards nervous breakdown can be arrested and reversed, no matter how far progressed. Panic attacks are often perpetuated because we instinctively handle them in the wrong way. The correct way of handling is elusive because it is somewhat counter intuitive. The panic attack feelings are so frightening that we tend to either try to escape them or we try to fight them. The key to success is to face and accept them instead. This should ring a bell, being the same treatment for fear. But Weeks has three more aspects to her calming method. And I can readily testify to their effectiveness.

First, when you face the symptoms, you should simply accept them. Initially this is breathtakingly hard to do. You are desperately short on spare energy to adopt such a mindset. Additionally, the symptoms cry out for some kind of remedial effort. They scream 'emergency' with an intensity that non-sufferers could not imagine. But instead, you should gently lower your reactivity to the situation, and simply observe the symptoms *without judgement*. In essence, meditate on them. If you fight them, you enflame them. If you judge them, your mind will jump to a plethora of scary conclusions, which will release more adrenaline and amplify them further.

Second, you should float. Just stay calm, with one eye casually and non judgementally observing the symptoms. Hard though it is to imagine when your heart is racing, and your breathing is spasmodic, that it is actually possible to relax. But, surprisingly, it is possible. This 'floating' relaxation will allow adrenaline and cortisol levels to lower.

Third, you should simply wait for the symptoms to subside. They are likely to do so in waves, and you should remain patient throughout. You should not expect the symptoms to disappear in a certain time. Let them take as long as they need to go. Being anxious about the time it takes will of course aggravate the symptoms once again.

It will take time and mental discipline to be able to apply these techniques, however, panic attacks fortunately tend to subside eventually on their own anyway. But it is best in the long term to be able to rid yourself of these attacks entirely. Note also that the patience required to see off one panic attack is also required long term, as panic attacks may persist, albeit at lower and lower levels for weeks, months or even years. Just like losing the fear that a dog will bite you takes time, so does ongoing persistence with panic attacks. Clare Weeks also makes the valid point that it does not serve you well to be self pitying. Subtly different from pity, however, self compassion will serve you well. Pity is a form of disgust, compassion a source of support. And if you do struggle supporting yourself, seek help from empathic others.

Sadly, in addition to the huge demand that panic attacks place on the sufferer, there is another layer of difficulty that often arises. The climax of fear that results in a panic attack can choose different forms of expression, making it hard to differentiate from a real, physical problem. There have been times when I have been convinced that I have been suffering with very low blood sugar, only to discover in hindsight that it was a mild panic attack, using uncomfortable low blood sugar symptoms as its means of expression.

Although you really do suffer badly if panic attacks blight your life, in addition to overcoming them, it is wise to treat them as individual ailments, and not see them as defining you. Suffering from panic attacks does not make you a weak person. To the contrary, it takes great strength to endure them. There is also the little matter that you never asked for them in the first place! They are simply part of your genetic heritage. Let who you are be defined by what you are, and not your experiences.

Chapter Twenty Two
You cannot control the World

Many have tried to control the world of course, not least evil men such as Hitler. His extraordinary, but barbaric attempts were, however, ultimately flawed. If you try to live a life that depends on controlling the world, you can set yourself up for a flawed existence. But many do persist in trying to live their lives like this. Many a marriage is headed for failure if each partner tries to change the behaviour of the other. Whilst humans *do* change, of course, expecting or coercing such change creates unhealthy attitudes. Your partner is likely to be treated as second best until they change. And we run the risk of keeping happiness in check until all the things in our life that need fixing are fixed – until we feel that *all* aspects of life have changed to suit our needs. As if that is ever likely to happen anyway!

The converse to the need for change is the acceptance of how things are, no matter how bad they might be. Sadly, most people stop before they even start to adopt an accepting attitude because they feel it is a passive, submissive approach to life. They fear that they will be downtrodden, unable to do *anything* about the things in life that annoy them.

But acceptance is very much *not* this. Acceptance is blindingly simple in its initial premise. Accept that the world, and you included, is the reality for you right in this moment. Accept that you have a stomach ache. Accept that the grass needs cutting. You should accept 'what is' because this is reality. Do not fight what is. Accept that you have just spilt your tea. But even accept that someone has just stolen your car?

Yes, because the key to acceptance does not end there, as many mistakenly believe. This first step is an *alignment with reality*. You accept that you have just discovered that your car is gone. You accept it because it has happened, and you cannot change that fact. However, acceptance does not leave you hopeless and helpless. It does not stop you then taking action. You should contact the police and ask neighbours if they saw anything. But by accepting what is, you do not fight reality. You are in harmony or synchrony with it. And the key benefit of acceptance here is that you do not complain about what has happened. Complaining will not reverse the situation, but will leave your brain in a negative frame of mind, as you seek retribution. Much better to accept and remedy the situation in the best way you can. In her book "Loving what is" on this subject, however, I feel that Byron Katie fails to embrace action, and is happy to let anarchy rule around her. LW

I should add an element of balance here. Whilst the more you can adopt an accepting attitude, the better, it can be very hard to accept adversity when you are overloaded by bad events. When the doorbell rings and your baby simultaneously starts screaming in the middle of cooking lunch, you can accept the situation, but you have precious little time or capacity to do deal with the reality of the situation. You must act, and will likely get stressed. Even then, however, if you can pause momentarily, you can seek to prioritise, turning the cooker down, and attending to your baby. The person at the door can wait for now. Better to do this than get highly flustered, where it is possible that you might leave your lunch to boil over as you rush to answer the door, shouting at the baby to be quiet on the way. Letting your emotions flare – getting angry at the overload – without accepting reality calmly and giving yourself a moment to prioritise will often serve you badly.

Before I go deeper into the concepts and benefits of an accepting mindset, I want to add my own caveat to the picture. As I studied acceptance and started applying it to my life, I noticed that the self help books tended to gloss over the relationship between acceptance, worry and action. After accepting something that we do not like, there are three basic scenarios :

1.   The thing we dislike is something we cannot or should not change.
2.   The thing we dislike is something we can change, should change, and know how to change.
3.   The thing we dislike is probably something that is possible to change, but we currently do not know how to change.

For number 1, acceptance allows us to let go of trying to make the change. You just accept it and move on in life. You should not worry about it because it is beyond your remit to do anything about. For number 2, we should focus on making the change, rather than on how much we dislike the problem as it stands now. If we procrastinate, and worry about the dislike, we fuel the discomfort accompanying the dislike. For example, a toothache may bug us for days, but as soon as we have booked a dental appointment, we can relax. We have taken action.

It is with number 3 that I have difficulties. My headaches fall into this category. I can and do accept my headaches, but they are still not yet banished from my life. There are things that I can yet try – I can and do take action – but after 16 years I am still trying. I cannot put all my efforts into fixing them because many approaches that I might take cost money and take time – time lost in treatment that then stops me earning the money to finance that treatment. And a focus on fixing my headaches tends to make me think of them more and thereby amplify them. So my conclusion with this ongoing type of concern is to see that any attempt at resolution is most likely to create a compromise, and therefore you should not get too caught up with the degree of your efforts to resolve the problem. But you should of course take periodic action to try to resolve the problem. Finally, and crucially, when not working on a resolution, you should stop worrying about the unresolved matter.

The key to all these things is to stop focusing on your dislike, injury, illness, or whatever, by first accepting it, and then taking action if and when this is appropriate. This therefore avoids the repeated and entrenched *worrying* that can follow from a repeated focus on the problem. Avoiding unnecessary worry is good for your health. We should either take action, plan for action if not immediately possible, or take no action now if appropriate not to. There should be no room for worry, since worry is a call to action. If we take action, the worry is being satisfied. If we cannot act, then we should defuse the worry. If we have to defer action, we can also defuse the worry because we have taken action to determine *when* to take action – any time spent worrying before then is pointless.

All well and good in theory, so how does this work in practice? For a few months now I have adopted the concept and moved from an almost perpetual state of worrier or anxiety to a much more free flowing, liberated state. You *can* change, as I have, by using this way of thinking to better handle opportunities for worry.

There is a saying about accepting your plight that you are quite likely to know :

*"It is not **what** happens to you that matters, but how you **react** to what happens to you that matters."*

I will rephrase this proverb a little :

*"It is not what happens to you that matters, but how your **conscious mind** reacts to how your **subconscious mind** reacts to what happens to you that matters."*

This is somewhat long-winded, but the point here is that our 'reaction' to something is not a neat, encapsulated thing, but more a series of interrelating events, starting with an initial and rapid assessment of the event by the emotion centres in your brain. Our lumbering conscious mind is given this emotional assessment in the form of a *colouring* of the actual event. For one personality type, the conscious mind is given a calm, measured picture of reality by their subconscious. In another type, the colouring is in the form of a heightened emotional state. The latter predisposes the conscious mind to be less rational about the event. The appearance of the same event to the conscious mind of different people can vary enormously by virtue of this initial emotional assessment by the emotional centres in their brain.

If you can recognise that these emotional flavourings to your perception of reality are making life hard, you should look to detach from them – to reduce how much you accept your subconscious mind's initial evaluation of situations. For example, if you get anxious, with a heightened heart rate when you see someone who you do not always get on with, then this may help you avoid them. But it actually may be your conscious desire to get on better with this person. So you should allow the emotions to calm down and not engage with them. Try to visualise a great conversation with them instead before you start talking with them.

Another aspect of acceptance is that you free yourself from regrets, and go more with the flow. You do not live in the past. You do not, for example, live in that moment when wine was split on your skirt. You move on. Complaining anchors you in the past.

It is worth repeating that acceptance does not mean submission. Paradoxically, by initially calmly accepting what is happening, rather than going into a rage, you can seek a more appropriate and valuable response. One that is less likely to damage relationships, or your health. Simply reacting to your initial gut response can lead you in the wrong direction. You might shout at your son for bumping into you, which caused you to spill your tea. If you had accepted that he had bumped into you before you react, you are more likely to calmly explain to him how tea can stain clothes and burn skin. By speaking calmly to him, he is more likely to take heed of what you say, and maybe learn a lesson, rather then feel the need to defend himself from a torrent of angry words.

There is a more subtle aspect to the acceptance philosophy. The concept of *pausing* so as to be more aware of the world around us. [RA] If you are in an accepting mind set when you pause, you will start to see things *as they are*. Often, we walk around in a slightly defensive mindset, looking to avoid bumping into people we would prefer not to speak to. This transfers into a more general failure to be fully receptive to everything around us. If you can walk along the street and accept all that you see without judgement, you will start seeing beauty in the simplest and most unexpected things. I remember vividly coming out of the cinema a few months ago, having been fortunate enough to see a heart-stirring film, where the rich colours portrayed in some scenes had a powerful emotional effect upon me. As I walked along the night-time roads, I found myself much more aware than normal of the brilliant colours of street and car lights and the breathtaking inky black of the background. This drew me into seeing details in buildings, as if I were a child again. An adult will see *some* buildings, but a child will see *these* buildings, with all their uniqueness, and this is how I felt. I paused to observe all the details around me in a kind of relaxed but very conscious trance. I felt free from judgement of what I saw, and free from the judgements of those around me, who might well have seen my behaviour as slightly odd, as I stopped every few moments to look more closely at something. At anything. Because all I saw seemed equally marvellous. Far better for me to enjoy the mesmerising pleasure of simple details than to worry about how I looked to others.

When it comes to our dark side, acceptance has a lot to offer. It is not your fault that you inherit the so-called 'negative' emotions such as anger, shame and disgust. By fighting them, or rejecting them, you do yourself no good. By accepting them, you are in line with reality. You **do** get angry if needed. You **can** get jealous of others. This is your genetic inheritance. By accepting this 'dark' side, and not pushing it away, you can start to accept yourself holistically. And you can start to relax, not apologising for yourself. Again, and this is crucial, accepting has to be accompanied by the responsibility for handling the *impact* of your dark side. But by no longer seeing the dark side as defining you (since you did not choose to have the capacity for these dark emotions in the first place), the health of your self-esteem is not dependant on avoiding these emotions, allowing you instead to handle them in a more relaxed, objective manner.

As Tara Brach neatly explained in her book "Radical Acceptance" [RA]:

> *"Our habit of being a fair-weather friend to ourselves - of pushing away or ignoring whatever darkness we can - is deeply entrenched."*

Accepting others for what they are also means accepting that they also have a dark side. They too are not guilty for what they have inherited genetically. The dark side is an appendage, and does not define them, just as it does not define you.

Likewise, choosing to accept pain rather than dull it is sensible, as I have already mentioned. But there is a spin on this, in that not only do most of us have a natural aversion to pain, but we get to see pain as an enemy. We get to hate coming down with a cold, rather than seeing it as a natural part of life. [RA] Suffering is part and parcel of life. When you start accepting that, you relax about life and start to take it in your stride. Stop fighting your cold and you will likely heal faster. Easier said than done, of course, as it can take a lot of mental discipline to accept suffering, but it is normally worth all the effort. By accepting this other dark side of life, you lower your defences, and lowered defences mean a healthier life.

Fundamentally, life is not fair, nor is it meant to be fair. This reality alone is reason enough to adopt acceptance as a philosophy. Work around problems, and injustices, and try to turn them to your advantage rather than dwell on them, and moan about them. As a programmer using the language Delphi back in 2002, I struggled to get to grips with its syntax and range of function. The documentation was frankly dire. So I saw this as an opportunity to write my own documentation, recording it on a web site (www.delphibasics.co.uk) for others to also use. I literally wrote the web site as I learnt the language. In light of the difficulties I had had, a high priority was for the site to be very easy to use for others. This was of course a rather large work around for the problem I had had with the dire Delphi product documentation!

But the web site proved popular enough to earn me a regular income, and eventually contact from Borland, the corporation that produced Delphi at the time. Danny Thorpe, then chief architect of Delphi emailed a request to me to extend my site to add an additional set of reference information regarding the new '.Net' component of Delphi. He had grown frustrated at the reluctance of his employers to match my level of documentation. How strange that a corporation can be surpassed by a single person. (Of course, the corporation was more interested in adding the functionality that was seen as a more likely magnet for potential purchasers).

Dealing with problems need not be this convoluted of course, but conceding defeat is often the wrong approach to take. Accept that there is a problem, but take action to resolve it if its resolution is important to you.

One final point on acceptance, on a rather sensitive subject – the acceptance of others who look or behave differently from ourselves. Millions of years of human existence has cultivated a strong defence of those genetically close to ourselves. Our parents and siblings are those we tend to protect, defend, and equate and side with most keenly. Cousins and second cousins share fewer genes, and we support them to an appropriately lesser degree. Because we are also tribal creatures, we also forge close bonds to friends and the groups we work and socialise with. By corollary, we tend to separate ourselves instinctively from other 'tribes' – other families and groups. But most of all, we seem heavily predisposed to instinctively reject those that differ most from ourselves.

It is taboo to say so, but a general truth to admit, that most of us find it easier to equate with people of like skin colour, intelligence, interests, styles of clothing, religious outlook, morals and so on. Much of this prejudice is innate, and largely genetically driven – we want to protect and propagate our genes, so gravitate towards people like ourselves.

But we should accept that most others are very different from ourselves. And that this different way that they live their lives is often their way of handling their own genetic heritage and circumstances – they are often doing the best they can, even if it differs from how we choose to live our lives. Many people find this aspect of acceptance particularly hard. But persevere and you can use the intellect to override your genetic urges, and ease away any prejudice against difference.

One of my favourite hobbies is to embrace in warm conversation any person I have an instinctive aversion to. It might be someone with too many ear, nose and tongue ornaments – a pet dislike of mine – or maybe someone with a really miserable countenance. At the food market I attend on Saturday mornings, the lady on one food counter is often indeed far from happy in demeanour, making me as a customer feel somewhat awkward. So I chatted with her one day, asking her if she was struggling with the cold without gloves. Within a few moments, her face broke out into a warm smile, and I was able to see another side of her, one that I had not seen before, and more likely her normal self when wrapped up warm at home. Often, you see, we make judgements without any chance of seeing the full picture.

Another day, I spotted a man sat on a long seat that I was passing on my way out of another film at the cinema. I gave him a big smile, and he duly smiled back. As I walked towards the escalator, I turned to see his face still beaming. And as I rode the escalator down to the ground floor, his smile was accompanied by a wave. I was able to connect with someone who I initially spurned by virtue of his appearance. And of course, the cultivation of this slightly odd habit – to accept all that I see around me – is both enlightening and a source of personal growth. The more I embrace the world, the easier it becomes.

I discussed this matter to a friend recently and made the observation as we spoke that many people, myself included, walk along the streets with blinkers on. We have our guard raised in response to the flood of people we are walking past and along with. So I try now to engage eye contact with random people as I walk. Doing so makes me realise not only quite how much I avoid eye contact, but also how much every one else does likewise. It is like a social taboo to embrace all around us. Yet we can do this. If you think back to times on holiday abroad, when you tend to embrace life and people in a very accepting way. True, we are relaxed and in no rush, but we are able to drop the defensive posture that blights our normal daily lives far too much. We look people in the face more, and chat more freely.

In the previous chapter, I described problems that I have with expectation, and how deviations were hard to handle. Expectation is a kind of control issue. We expect life to go a certain way and suffer angst when it does not. It is best to have a flexible outlook, and not get emotionally attached to expectations. One of my regular expectations is to be able to make the most of the rare sunshine we get in the UK. If a week of rainy weather is followed by hot sun on the very day that I have to be stuck indoors, I can become glum, and complain about the unfairness of it all. This and anger are common consequences of unmet expectations. SE Better for me to accept the situation and invest my energies in that situation. Better for my mind to be where my body was rather than for my mind to be where my body evidently was not.

Perfectionism is a form of expectancy. It expresses itself as an over sensitivity to flaws in what we or others do. This expectation of flawless performance is best moderated to allow for some slack, in order to better handle less than perfect outcomes. It is not so much that perfectionism is unachievable, but more that it is often not needed, and indeed very often expensive or even impossible to attain.

Curiously enough, the ten years I spent as an amateur cabinet maker were mostly devoid of perfectionist tendencies, right from day one. I do not quite know why this was the case, but I do remember appreciating the freedom to produce that this gave, liberated from the constraint of frequent critical self appraisals. In ten years of amateur carpentry, I completed all but 2 projects (time ran out before I moved house), and was never called upon to explain shortcomings in my work. Even when I pointed out flaws, the customer was often none the wiser. It helped of course that wood is a very accommodating material, and tended to show the glory of its patina with only a little effort on my part, but a perfectionist approach is often out of line with how the rest of the world sees or expects things.

By avoiding the fear of making mistakes, I was able to propel myself in all sorts of directions, exploring my creativity, rather than fussing over little flaws. The fear of making mistakes can be like a straight jacket. I remember one day when inlaying some final pieces of veneer into a large chess-board, my arm accidentally knocked over a plastic bottle of glue. It poured all over the newly laid veneer. I do not think I even swore. I remember that I simply accepted the situation – it was indeed too late to change what had happened – and scooped up as much glue as I could back into the container. A dull wet mark was left on the veneer, and I just assumed that it would not penetrate very far. This was a somewhat optimistic judgement since veneers are only 0.5 mm thick! As it happens, my lack of fussing was justified – the sanding down process went right through the wet layer. I sanded away all evidence of my mishap, and a fine chessboard came through this ordeal. If I had fussed and become upset, I would have failed to enjoy the hard toil of the sanding process, or maybe even have lifted the veneer and started over in a less than happy frame of mind.

Many of us are held back from enjoying life, from being happy, by an inverse form of expectation. We think that we cannot possibly expect to be happy until our health is sorted, the mortgage is paid off, we get our dream job, and that injury heals. Such a negative expectation predicated on events or things will in its nature ensure its own perpetuation. As soon as one 'key criteria' for enjoying life is ticked off, the next item in the list kicks in. But meanwhile, we encounter a new stream of events or projects that will be deemed to equate with unhappiness or impaired life quality until ticked off. So they get added to the list and the list never ends.

A few months ago, I started suffering strange problems in my legs. The details are irrelevant, but the problem was a source of great worry, not least because each route I explored on the Internet seemed to lead to bad news. I love walking and soccer too much to face such a prospect. So my life was on hold until the problem was fixed. Until I decided otherwise. I chose to start accepting whatever fate was in store for my poor legs. I would start from this day onwards to enjoy life. To go with the flow as much as possible and simply enjoy wherever it took me. Sure, I had plans, and soccer was a major part of those plans. But I decided then to make my plans with a flexible attitude. I would twist and bend and reroute as needed, and try not to complain. This tendency to complain has often been a big part of my nature, driven by strong emotions. But it rarely helped fix matters. Instead, I decided to accept what might happen. I even visualised a worse case scenario of amputation and accepted what that might bring. Paradoxically, I realised, it might possibly get more me attention in a wheelchair than I currently get as an able bodied person, and consequently possibly even more time to spend writing.

Recently, I waited in until mid afternoon for the arrival of a new cable TV box. An upgrade to my existing box, with extra bells and whistles of course. Two and a half hours after it had arrived, with much time on the telephone to the cable company support department, it not only transpired that the new box had a fault, but that I could not revert to using my old box. The failed activation process for my new box was a one-way process, it seems. They had not allowed for the possibility that a new box might not work, so I would have to wait until the next afternoon before an Engineer could come out to help me. Which meant that I was unable to watch the big soccer match on TV that evening.

Of course, you would assume that I would have said to the support staff something like "I am not exactly happy about this!" But I didn't. Nor did I think of saying it. I had decided all through this that I would not let the new box (a material thing) or the missing of the TV programme (an event thing) affect how I felt. I just went with the flow. There was nothing more that the support department could do, so I accepted my plight, and relaxed in the sun. And as I relaxed there, I realised that I felt very happy.

You might be wondering why on earth I should have felt so happy. I had paid for something that had not worked. I was going to miss my soccer match. And I had wasted over 2 hours to get to that position. I was happy because of *how I had handled* these problems. I was happy not because of some material thing. I was happy not because of some event. I was happy because of the resilience and flexibility of my attitude. For most of my life, I would have suffered negative emotions with such an unfortunate sequence of events. And you can rightly guess that even if it was possible, I would be unlikely to arrange for such a sequence of events to transpire in the future in order to reap the happiness benefits. I do believe that this confirms the opinion I voiced earlier that happiness is a consequence of attitude, and not something that can be forced into existence.

To expect life to be just right before you can truly enjoy it is one of the biggest mistakes most of us make. It does not help of course that we are not taught the fault in such a way of thinking. But at least you now know. And if you buy into this idea, you will amaze yourself with what transpires. Some days, I just look up at the trees and say 'I am alive', and think that in all the billions of years this planet has been here, and will be here, I am indeed here, alive, in my tiny slot of time. And I appreciate life more by doing this. I live in the moment. And yes, research has shown that the more you live in the moment, accepting all that is around you, the happier you will be, and the longer and healthier your life will be.

At the end of the day, expectations are, of course, a product of the ego, a controlling force in the mind, and this is where I will be taking you in the next chapter.

Chapter Twenty Three

Ego

The famous psychologist Sigmund Freud developed a 3 part structure of the human psyche. The **Id** covered the basic unconscious drive for pleasure and the avoidance of pain. The **Ego** was designated as a partially conscious component which seeks to satisfy the Id in the long term for a person, striking a balance between immediate Id needs and the ongoing welfare of that person. The **Super-ego** was designated as the mostly unconscious component of our psyche which seeks to make us live in an idealistic way, often contradicting the primitive Id needs.

Because the ego is linked to, and driven by the primitive needs that are a large part of our genetic inheritance, it is often at odds with our intellect and with modern life. The Super-ego tries to compensate, but it is often better for us if we try to release the grip of the ego on our lives. Not that this is a simple matter of course, nor is it possible to be completely free from primitive drives of the ego. They have indeed served us well for millions of years of course. But the advent of the higher brain functions in homo sapiens allows us to keep the ego in check. If we choose to. Sadly, most people do not even realise that they are under ego-control, or that such control can be relinquished. Instead, they succumb to many raw emotions that tend to drive and rule their existences.

One outcome of the ego's grip on our lives is that most people have a vague ongoing feeling of discontentment. ™ Our ego regularly nags us to buy things, thereby engaging in a cycle of material acquisition, novelty, familiarity and then boredom that drives us to new acquisitions for their novelty – for the next 'fix'. And we fail to spot this pattern, even though it can persist throughout our lives. Our ignorance of the demands and influence of the ego is a kind of delusion. We end up obsessing to have that which we do not have, and to be that which we are not. We are perpetually driven by a sense that the grass is greener elsewhere.

There is a value in this restlessness however. It coerces us to explore and engage in life. It makes us get out and engage in new experiences. But it does so in the wrong way, leaving us in a state of discontentment for much of the time. We feel anxious seeking out and obtaining a new thing or experience, and fail to enjoy the journey. We place too much value on achievement rather than in the *process* of achievement. And expectation can dull enjoyment as well. If we release the ego, we live more lightly, more in the moment – enjoying the journey, even if we find the shop is shut. Capitalism thrives on, and amplifies our discontentment. It really does not want us to be content. After buying the state of the art digital camera this year, we are made to feel that it is woefully inadequate next year when it is superceded by a 'superior' model.

I alluded to this in the last chapter, when I described how I let go of the need to wait for life to be perfect before I could be happy. In essence, I was letting go of my ego, which insisted that I could not be content without continually satisfying its never ending stream of needs and wants. The ego is possessive – it always wants – like a perpetual child within us. But these needs and wants do not have to define who we are. The ego is essentially dysfunctional by nature, and we should reduce its power over us. [RA]

We can indeed release ourselves from this ego-driven lifestyle. And yes, like many changes I recommend, this is not easy, requiring the expected determination and a sustained concentration of effort. This is in part because the ego is devious and will find many ways to reinstate its supremacy. For example, if you adopt some of the concepts in the next chapter, and selflessly start doing favours for others, the ego will kick in asking us to make sure we get our 'entitlement' of a return favour. But this largely defeats the purpose of selflessness. So you have to remain ever vigilant, on the look out for the elusive ways of the ego. Even those who achieve great success with spiritual enlightenment can find the ego pushing them to tell everyone how well they are doing with their enlightenment!

The achievement of status in modern life is a common aspiration, but it too is often overly driven by the ego, forcing us to aspire to status without seeing the consequences. The ego distorts our balance. Much as the drive for profit and growth can blind corporations to some of the negative impacts they can have on many people. The ego can obsess so much about matters such as status that it can even cause the break up of friendships 'which get in the way of success', and even to the break up of marriages.

Note, as an aside, that the attraction of status drives us both to acquire it and to seek out attachments with those who already have it. These attachments probably evolved through the centuries as an advantageous strategy – the power of social bonds with the rich, famous and successful often results in benefits coming our way. This is evident in the matter of employment – most job placements are made via social networks rather than by job interviews.

Taoism (pronounced Day-oh-isum) is a set of mostly philosophical Chinese traditions going back to around 500 B.C. The principle writing on the subject is "Tao Te Ching" by Las-Tzu, translated into English by Arthur Wayle in 1934 as "The Way and its Power". The three basic components of Taoism are moderation, humility and compassion. Moderation and humility can only really be achieved by a subordinance of the ego. Compassion is covered in the next chapter.

Taoism also concerns itself with a global energy that is claimed to pervade all and everything. Matter is made of energy, and because the atmosphere we breath and move around in is made of matter, we are in effect swimming in a sea of energy. Taoism wants us to tap into this energy that connects us all. By doing so, we become more alive and connected to a power much greater than ourselves. I personally have a bit of a struggle with such concepts, but at least Taoism also has offers wisdom that supports the refocusing away from ourselves, and in particular from our ego, so is valuable for these matters alone. In its extreme form, Taoism teaches us to let go so much that our personality itself becomes less well defined. This is a hard concept to grasp, let alone attain. You might be able to see that the common desire to have a well defined personality is yet another manifestation of ego possessiveness. I told you that it was pervasive.

It appears that tapping into this 'infinite' energy source cannot be forced. There may be evidence here of some religious throwbacks in Taoism, as you must let the energy guide you, and not try to control it, much as you are meant to give yourself fully to the Christian God as your guiding force. With Taoism, you let the energy within you manifest itself.

If you let the ego control you, it projects outwardly as it seeks to satisfy its needs. What is projected outward generally gets reflected back. If we are greedy, we see greed in others. Project warmth and warmth is more likely to be reflected back. But the ego is not terribly excited by this softly softly approach, and will look to see what it can get out of the process. You must be forever on your guard!

Successfully connecting with this mass of energy takes much repeated practice. Both the ego and the influence of negative people can compromise your efforts. [WL] However, if you cannot avoid the company of negative people, try to understand life from their perspective and try to see them as teachers. Learn from the damage that negativity has inflicted upon them. And maybe try to help them also.

As you detach from the ego, you will start to detach from both a need for material things and also for routine. The ego is very keen on routine, so one way of releasing its grip is to forge a habit for doing things differently. Break up your routines. Research has show that even two weeks of doing two things a day differently from normal elevates happiness levels, much to the surprise of the participants.

Friends, family and work will continue to both condition your behaviour and put expectations upon you. As you release the grip of your ego and become less attached to needs and routines, you will likely find that you accede less and less to their demands. You will not so much adopt an anarchic position as no longer play the same social games that the ego in those around you is imploring you to embrace. And of course, you might lose some 'friends' along the way. Any true friend , however, will hopefully see that you are not hell bend on an anti-social journey, but one of personal growth, and elect to hang in there with you, eventually seeing the benefits.

Ok, this may all sound a bit scary and contrived. But if I explore the matter of morals, you will at least start to see how releasing the ego can make us more morally consistent and more rational about morality.

Our morals are a mix of behaviours and attitudes that we assign with good and bad labels. We put such a high value on our morals that we are very careful to pick and choose friends who most closely match them. Yet we delude ourselves into thinking that we have got the mix right. [IR] That these behaviour and attitude mixes vary so much from person to person should give you a clue that the majority of us must have flaws in our choice of mix. These different moral mixes cannot all be right. Yet we are arrogant enough to believe that our own personal mix is better than others. And guess what drives this arrogance?

Much more insidious is how often we break our own moral codes, yet heavily criticise others for doing so. We are fundamentally inconsistent, yet are mostly too delusional to notice. For example, many people have the sensible social moral not to steal from others. Yet research has shown that very few with this moral always see stealing for what it is. Shopkeepers in a number of shops agreed to participate in an experiment where excess change was given to customers. When a customer paid for something costing less than £5, and used a £5 note, the shopkeeper was instructed to give change as if he had been given a £10 note. Few people handed back the excess change. Even allowing for those who simply failed to spot the error, many were knowingly leaving the shop with money that was not theirs to take, in effect stealing from the shopkeeper. The moral not to steal had lost its potency because the situation did not fit the moral picture – the customer did not *instigate* the theft – it was a fault of someone else. Curiously, the number of people handing back the excess change was much higher when they had shopped in a small, local shop. In a big retail chain shop, returns were much lower. We are, it seems, happy to be flexible as well as inconsistent in the meaning of our morals – we feel that the big shop can afford to lose the odd £5, but the corner shop cannot.

In their book "Take me to truth", Sanchez and Vieria describe a multi-stage process for undoing the ego. ™ It is worth noting that these stages do not run smoothly from start to finish. The release of the ego is something of a rollercoaster ride, as we experience instability without it – for good or bad, our ego has been a lifelong companion, and is necessarily reluctant to go lose its power. As we loosen the ego grip, we move out of the comfort zones that the ego has furnished for us. The ego fades away in cycles, reemerging at times in a kind of death throw.

For many people, the effort required to navigate this ego release path can only come from a position of great need, such as when they have reached rock bottom in life. Because they have become so ill or destitute, they will have experienced such devastation that the hardship entailed in quelling the influence of the ego is a much smaller task. If they choose the Taoist path to a better life, their rock bottom starting point makes them extremely determined to succeed.

Letting go of the ego allows you to gain flexibility in life. To go with the flow. To suffer pain without complaint. The ego normally resists pain, of course. It also resists change that comes from a flexible lifestyle. It resists the discomfort of the unknown. By moving from a life of resistance to one of flexibility, we are liberated, and in greater health.

The subconscious chatterbox that I have already mentioned is often driven by the ego. Rather than buy into all it has to say, try instead to listen to your intuition. The chatter is a stream of commentary about the world around us. Or more accurately, the attempt by the ego tainted subconscious to understand the world. According to research, much of this understanding is flawed and compounded by misguided projections into the future. LW Indeed, the ego prefers to lie to us rather than face some of the harsh realities of the world (optical illusions are a simple demonstration of this). It is also uncomfortable with incomplete knowledge – this fear of the unknown – and fills in the gaps rather than give us incompleteness. This leads to such mental problems as the CBT mind-reading and forecasting habits many of us have.

Do not let your chatterbox define who you are. When you start to understand that your stream of thoughts are often faulty and ego driven, you can live more in the conscious mind – you can let the higher functions in the brain rule in place of low-level functions like the ego and emotions. The chatterbox, it should be pointed out, is relentless, judging, forecasting, complaining and wanting. [IS]

After years spent on the receiving end of the chatterbox, the ego's distorted view of the world will have an accumulating effect . You are likely to have developed generalisations about the world and its people that are often crude and unhealthy. And these generalisations can stop you seeing reality for what it is.

If we buy into negative thoughts from the ego, we serve only to legitimise them, and they become a bigger reality, swamping out positive thoughts. The ego is :

"... like a weed that eventually chokes you to death." [IS]

Conversely, buying into positive thoughts enhances them. They become our reality. [EB]

To start to get the feel of both the power of the grip of the ego and of what it takes to release that grip, there are exercises you can carry out. They push you outside of the comfort zone that the ego wants you to be a permanent resident of. Try walking in the pouring rain next time without any thought of complaint. Remove your hat and feel the rain pound on your head, and then trickle down you neck. It is surprisingly liberating. Pouring rain on a Saturday morning normally deters around half of my friends from turning up to the afternoon game of soccer. Yet if the rains come down after 10 minutes of play, we all carry on regardless. So banishing the ego's comfort grip is eminently possible.

A more interesting exercise is to wear a blindfold for a few hours, forcing you to navigate around your house by fumbling. [IS] You experience great discomfort initially, but it is unexpectedly empowering after an hour or so – the ego has blinded us to some of the possibilities that come from extending beyond our comfort zones like this.

The Taoist way is not just about the suppression of the ego. It is also very much about humility, and living the honourable life. [15] For many, this will sound like an old fashioned idea, not suited to modern life. I agree that it is lifestyle choice that has been mostly forgotten, but I believe that it is worth resurrecting for your own benefit as much as it is for the benefit of others. A cornerstone of an honourable life is honesty towards others and, crucially, towards yourself. And, yes, both of these forms of honesty are very difficult to achieve. But a coherent attitude towards honesty in all spheres of your life is wonderfully invigorating. It also has a simplifying effect on your social life.

If you choose to adopt an attitude of honesty, you will necessarily struggle to cast off life long habits that you were not fully aware you had. And you will likely suffer social difficulties. 'Does my bottom look big in this?' is indeed very hard to answer honestly. Tact in social matters is a glue that helps stick us together. But such matters are essentially at the tip of the iceberg. Much deeper is the less frivolous face you show to others. Does your sweet, friendly manner hide ulterior motives? Ask yourself if you do favours to others as a part of of a social creed where a return of the favour is expected? Are you being honest with yourself about your own intentions? Are you being honest with others in doing favours with the right heart, or doing favours as a subtle form of manipulation that seeks their approval of you?

Our hidden motives are often spotted by others, and they can then become wary of our intentions. Trying to see our own motives – to be honest in the *intent* behind our actions – is hard to do, but one that can be acquired with practice. Do you really give to charity to help those in need, or is it more likely that you are doing it to look good? Do you open a door for someone to help them through, or for the thanks your action should solicit? Do you give up your seat in a bus to look superior to those who have not done so? These ulterior motives spring from the ego, and a focus on honesty is a further way to release its grip.

Being honest to yourself and being honest to others also means being honest *about* yourself to others. Admitting, without being asked, that you were guilty in some endeavour that undermined a group effort is a form of active honesty that is hard to master. The instinct of the ego is to keep quiet about our failing and hope that things die down. However, doing 'what you can get away' sows a seed of devious behaviour that can come back to haunt you. It is a form of passive dishonesty. A dishonesty of attitude.

Being honest about someone in their absence is likewise tough to do. Whilst it is much better not to talk ill of someone in their absence, if conversation does move to such a topic, I will try to personally respect the person in their absence. If the absent person were to walk in, I hope that I would not change what I had to say. I would hope to be as true in my words talking *to* them as I would talking *about* them in their absence.

I recently had the good fortune to chat with an overtly friendly couple in a nearby bar. It transpired that she was a reflexologist, and believed that my tension headaches might benefit from reflexology treatment. That it helps her own tension headaches gave me reason to consider trying out this line of therapy. I openly admitted that my headaches were not a problem these past few weeks – the more engrossed I had become in my writing, the less headaches had impacted my days. But that if and when they returned, I would arrange an appointment.

We all say such things. But we mostly use this deferral device to avoid making a commitment there and then. But I now try to follow through with my honesty. If I say that I will contact her when I am again blighted by headaches means that I *will* contact her (as long as my unreliable memory enables me). I try to be honest with my commitments to others. And I really can assure you that the burden of doing so is more than offset by the feeling of integrity that it generates. Being able to say things to people, *knowing* that you will follow through makes your words truly authentic. Others can pick up on the subtle cues you give when you fail to communicate authentically. Of course, I have to be sure that I want to commit, so I will also be honest if I know that I will not want to follow on. I will not give false hopes.

The discipline required to be honest not only becomes a discipline towards commitments to others. It also extends to discipline towards yourself. If you said to yourself that you would make sure the front room would be tidy before the end of the weekend, then make sure it happens. Sticking to personal commitments is empowering. It also strengthens your self esteem. Succumbing to the ego's desire to 'chill out' rather than meet an obligation will instead serve only to perpetuate your tendency to procrastinate. Fighting procrastination can be a long tough battle, but the rewards, yet again, are immense.

Wherever possible, pay your debts. Both the financial ones and the social ones.

Treat people fairly, without using your judgement of them, or their weaknesses as a means of manipulating them.

Being honest in all endeavours does not mean that you have to agree to all requests. It does not mean that you have to be a soft touch (although being compassionate and kind is fine). If you do not want to do something where there is a genuine choice not to, means that you should say that you will not. If you cannot do something with the right attitude, but agree to do so, you are more likely to find yourself doing it for the wrong reasons, often seeking compensation for your begrudging efforts.

As I have mentioned already, being honest is liberating, even if it is hard to feel the liberation at first. But it also means that you grow in confidence about yourself. You stop hiding from yourself or others. You acquire a greater coherency of behaviour. Others trust you more, knowing that when you agree to do something, you will always do it, and do so willingly, with no hidden need for a return favour. If someone abuses such innocent giving, then you will find after a while that you will not want to give to that person, and so will start saying no to their requests. These rebuttals will more likely make them start appreciating you than become a source of irritation that you 'let them down'. Conversely, if you always agree to the requests of others, you are likely to be taken for granted. DP

The key here is not to arbitrarily stop helping others, but to help only when you genuinely want to (or have to), and where the help is appreciated and warranted.

Finally, it is worth reminding you that the ego's interminable drive for 'more' often blinds you to what you already have. If you pause and respect the food on your plate, the roof over your head, your friends and family, it will give you a much better perspective on the cloying needs of the ego.

The final Taoist focus is on moderation. You can avoid overindulgence by eating slowly, by enjoying what you have without a constant gaze at the greener grass elsewhere. By consuming to excess, you create an expectancy of the same in the future. Moderation in most things, most of the time, is key to a balanced and healthy life – and means that the harmless odd overindulgence is truly savoured.

Chapter Twenty Four

Compassion and kindness

Moving away from the demands of the ego allows you to start embracing your fellow man more, without seeking to gain from that embrace. You start to enjoy them for what they are, and not what you might gain from that friendship. It is a sad fact that the first time we meet someone, we tend to subconsciously assess what they can offer us. If you can release this ego-driven habit, you can start opening your heart and eyes to all that you meet. You will feel the pull of the ego, but letting that pull fade, and embracing them *for what they are* can be such a sweet experience. If you can look them in the face and see them *without any judgement at all* then you will enter a momentary state of deep relaxation, and be able to connect with them in an equally deep way. I assure you that most people will detect your openness. Most interpersonal interactions are influenced by fleeting facial expressions that our subconscious is very adept at detecting. We are not consciously aware of these observations – they serve as fragments of the picture being painted behind the conscious mind's awareness. But our subconscious will use such snippets to guide subsequent treatment of that person. They will influence the level of trust we might invest in that person. It is very much not what we say, but how we say it that matters, and even more how very much our attitude when speaking is expressed in our faces.

Accepting others is a starting point for compassion and kindness. Try to care for everyone you meet. Care for all that is around you – do not even kill insects simply because they irritate you. Much of the damage to the Earth is a consequence of a failure for compassion for other people, animals and the environment. Corporations are often an embodiment of anti-compassion. Their insatiable but unnecessary greed for growth and profit can blind them to human compassion. They are happy to earn money from drugs that are known to have serious side effects. They are happy to pollute rivers and cut swathes through Amazonian rain forests, regardless of the ecological consequences.

The converse that I am recommending, where we have a compassionate view of our fellow man and of the ground we stand upon, is an antidote to some of these big business ills. Whilst even the collective efforts of those who embrace compassion is unlikely to put a brake on the corporate juggernaut, it will have a significant bearing on our own health and that of others around us.

As part of the research for "The Plastic Mind", Sharon Begley visited Buddhist monks who practiced compassionate meditation. [PM] And that included the Dalai Lama. After decades of focusing on feelings of love and compassion for all people, an end product was not that they no longer had to suppress feelings like jealousy, or irritation. But that they were no longer able to *feel* these emotions. The repeated focus on compassion had completely emphasised positive emotions and de-emphasised negative emotions.

The world that we live in has sadly trivialised the power of compassion. In the words of Kahlil Gibran :

"Tenderness and kindness are not signs of weakness and despair, but manifestations of strengths and resolutions"

Paradoxically, it requires a strength of character to move away from personal needs to address the needs of, and be warm to, other people. Alas, much of modern life fuels the ego too much, where social cohesion is replaced by individual survival – we tend more and more to look after number one first. Yet this is in spite of the synergistic gains that the whole concept of society had brought to humans in the first place. We are in a sense destroying that which made us what we are. By returning to a society where we look out for each other, we all gain. Research has shown that belonging to communities is hugely beneficial to health. [CM]

But compassion, kindness, and the empathic consideration of others brings a more profound benefit. And it starts right at the beginning of human life. The development of the brain in babies and children is enormously affected by these factors. They act as a signal to the baby that the environment is safe and supportive. This allows the baby to develop in a more relaxed state of mind. Conversely, a harsh environment, where being attended to with love and compassion is rare or inconsistent, destines children to have more stunted physical growth, and a much greater tendency for a nervous disposition. The reaction shown here is a defensive response to an environment that is perceived to be hostile. The effect of these two extremes of upbringing have very long lasting effects. Children born into nurturing, loving environments are much more likely to be easy going in nature, more resistance to disease and generally healthier. [CM]

Compassion proffered to adults has a similar bearing on their health. Those adults who can feel assured of compassionate and supportive friends and family are most likely to be in good mental and physical health. Yet we live in a world where such compassion is almost frowned upon!

A significant failing of the medical profession is to underestimate the importance of compassion in the well being of patients. If they were to focus more on the holistic health of their patients, they would ensure that they were emotionally supported – to prioritise the patient perspective ahead of protocol. As Gilbert says :

"Medicine can prolong dying, which is not the same as prolonging life"

Compassion also crucially breeds more compassion. It is as much a kind of benevolent virus as the self-centred lifestyle that we seem coerced to follow is a malignant one. The act of caring for our fellow man, woman and child, of tolerating differences, and accepting failings without the need for retribution all fall under the compassion umbrella. Compassion can significantly offset some of the ills of modern life. It acts as a binding force, and the key strength of humans is their collective strength. The whole is greater than the sum of the parts.

If compassion for others is a rare event in modern times, then compassion for self is even rarer. If compassion and kindness for others is seen as a weakness and an unaffordable soft option in the cut and thrust of modern life, then such support turned inwardly is seen as nothing other than a form of narcissism, with all the connotations that that implies. Of course, there is a vast difference between caring for yourself in times of need and indulging your whims and fancies in spite of the needs of others around you. Compassion for self must also not be confused with pity. Pity is shame about oneself, as I have said before, and is best avoided.

Because of the negative associations of self-compassion, of images of self-indulgence, *many of us treat others better than we treat ourselves.* Only upon reflection can we start to realise the reality of this bizarre imbalance. And the concept of imbalance is an appropriate one to focus on. If we do not attend to (or allow others to attend to) our own needs enough, then we become too weak and tired and stressed to attend to the needs of others. I cannot over emphasise the importance of this aspect of self compassion. By giving time and space for healing for ourselves, we become more capable of helping others, whether that be in a family, friend or work situation.

Much as you should give yourself some slack for your genetic inheritance, so you should give yourself slack when you get tired, hungry, irritable or ill just as you would a close member of your family. If you have not given yourself time to rest, you will struggle to handle your discomfort and get negatively emotional. But if you have had the opportunity to be compassionate about yourself and rested, then the primitive emotional urge may not arise, or if it does, you will be able to handle it better. Be kind and compassionate towards yourself so that your health is preserved.

Taking compassion to a more proactive level, research shows that a few hours a week spent working for a charity, such as in one of their retail shops, is good both for the community and for your own well being. ᵂᴷ Helping others in the generic sense is good for the soul. It is a socially cohesive action, and a win-win activity, as long as, of course, it is done with the right attitude.

One key benefit that arises from helping others is of course a transference of focus away from ourselves. Kindness has been shown to elevate levels of endorphins, serotonin, dopamine and oxytocin. [WK] The last of these is described as a social hormone. Warmly hug someone, and oxytocin is released. The bond between mother and baby results in high levels of oxytocin.

One immediate consequence of elevated oxytocin levels is increased eye contact, enhancing intimacy and warmth. Compare with the commonly defensive stance most take, where eye contact is fleeting at most. Next time you engage in conversation, try to engage in more eye contact, and at the same time try to see how often the face of the person you are talking with is angled a little away from you. Too long ago to remember the source, alas, I recall reading about the effect of eye angle between two people. When eye contact is direct, very specific neural networks light up. It takes only a few degrees off axis to stop them firing. We are very highly influenced by the degree of directness of eye contact.

Oxytocin levels go through the roof in the early stages of love. [WK] We consequently embrace anything and everything around us. It has a hugely calming and forgiving effect on us. We see love all around. Oxytocin calms the amygdala down, so that we are less reactive to emotional stress. It even aids digestion, protects the heart and reduces inflammation. [WK]

Even if you are not naturally kind and giving, cultivating this outlook is indeed possible. Millionaires have been known to give up all and change their view on life as the penny dropped about some of the fundamental values in life that they had been blinded to in their thrust for wealth and status. We can change. Love and kindness to our fellow man, and an acceptance of the twists and turns that life offers us calms and relaxes us. We move from the common place habit of almost permanent defensiveness to one of acceptance, and warm engagement with all around us. There is also an evolutionary basis for warmth and kindness, as it fostered greater social bonding. Social coherence has synergistic benefits that make a social group much more powerful than the sum of its members. Here, our improved health improves the health of our community which then reflects back to us. Another virtuous cycle.

My own health policies

I have covered a vast amount of ground in this book, and I feel it would be valuable to provide two summary chapters. I do so because I believe that many may want to refresh their memories but do not have time to reread the whole book.

This first summary here is an illustration of how I have personally endeavoured to apply some of the principles I have offered here. I have cherry picked some concepts from this book and absorbed them into my own life in order to try to improve my health. It is crucial to note that I have not tried to adopt all of the ideas in the book.

First, it would require a super human effort to do this all in one go, or at all in fact. Releasing the grip of the ego, for example, can be a life-long challenge. Second, that good health is normally attainable by adjusting just a few aspects of your life – you really do not need to apply all of the suggestions offered. Focus on the key areas that you want to pick up on, and start to adopt them. If and when they become established parts of your life or personality, you can then add a few more health improving changes. By starting off in the right direction, there really is no need to rush, or to see your health as liable to failure or compromise if you do not accommodate all of the ideas presented.

I tried to strike a balance across the health spectrum. Here are the concepts that I have adopted in the last year or so.

1. A low carbohydrate diet

The impact that food cravings used to have on me whilst eating a *high* carbohydrate diet was very wearing. I could not choose when to eat – I had to eat little and often so as to avoid the worst of the blood sugar drops that I had suffered with for decades. Blood sugar yo-yoing that created mood swings as well. The adoption of a low-carbohydrate diet has proven to have had a major impact. By mostly eating just 3 fat-enriched, low-carbohydrate meals per days, I have many hours between each with a stability of blood sugar and therefore of mood that was previously totally alien to me.

After a year or so on the diet, I now, sadly, take it for granted. But occasionally when I do not eat quite the right balance of foods and go just a bit too long between meals, my hypoglycaemic symptoms return. Rather than feel slowly more hungry as meal time approaches – what I am now used to – the food craving caused by this rare instance of hypoglycaemia is a stark reminder of what I have thankfully left behind. For those who do not suffer low blood sugar, the transition from satiety to craving can be as little as 10 minutes. It is not so much that you are hungry, but more that the floor has fallen away from you. Your hunger appears bottomless, and you start to feel ill. You get light headed, weak, very irritable and obsessed by the need to eat.

It is hugely liberating to be mostly free from these unsettling and uncomfortable symptoms. To be able to slowly cook a meal 7 hours after breakfast and then eat without cramming food down fast is simply fantastic, even if it is normal for most people. That I lost weight on the diet was a neat bonus as well. Additionally, my headaches have faded mostly into the background, and on most days, I have a very high level of mental clarity.

2. Avoiding pharmaceutical products

Looking at last to follow in my father's footsteps, I now try to avoid taking any drugs at all. If I suffer pain, then I try to feel and accept it, and not hide it. I believe that this is starting to make me stronger. By taking aspirin, paracetamol or ibuprofen for example, I would merely dampen the awareness of my body, and leave myself open to the side effects of these drugs.

I guess that you are not surprised from what I have written in this book that I take a largely anti-pharma stance. And this means also that I have grown wary of the benefits that my doctor can offer me. That doctors now struggle to see patients as anything other than transporters of symptoms does not give me much confidence in their ability to help me in an appropriately holistic fashion, I am afraid.

3. Giving without expecting return

When I do a favour for someone now, I do so with a strong focus on suppressing any ulterior motives that might arise in my mind that seek compensation for my efforts. I also try to suppress any urge to complain about the degree of effort required to do the favour. I gave my nephew a lift to a sports day event yesterday, and on the way home, stuck in traffic, my subconscious badgered me to later tell my sister how much I was inconvenienced. This petty streak in my psyche is a part of my personality that I just have to accept. I do not like it, but by the same token, I do not choose to feel this way, so need not punish myself for the feelings. This is an instinct that does not serve me well, so I do not buy into it. I try to override it each time it manifests, and it grows weaker each time as a consequence.

4. Complaining less

Following on from the example above, I try really hard not to complain about things. The difficulty I have here is that I have very easily enflamed emotions, and candidate situations for complaint arise readily (much as situations of joy arise as prime topics for conversational anecdote). I do find it valuable to release the emotional tension from bad events, but now I try to do so with humour, releasing the angst in a way that flavours future memories of the event with a lighter, more positive taste. By reframing this way, I set up a positive habit, making it much more likely that future 'traumas' are swiftly seen with a jovial hindsight. And eventually, I hope to be able to laugh at a trauma as it happens. Well, at least, that is my aim.

5. Focus on life and not on problems

Avoiding the urge to complain about something, or to reframe when I have to tell of my plight, is to move focus away from the negativity within that something. Generalising this further, I now look to focus my attention on living life, and not on the problems and suffering that is an expected part of life. This change of focus was made much easier by my bourgeoning habit of avoiding the urge to complain.

By changing my focus in life, I am training my attention. What we pay attention to becomes our reality. It makes entire sense to focus on positive things rather than negative. What we focus on becomes a locus. This touches on the recently very popular concept generally known as the 'Law of Attraction'. When we focus on positive things, this very process not only makes our mind attract positive memories, but appears to have an effect on the rest of the world. I leave it up to you to explore this interesting topic. But it is not so implausible that the world essentially brings positive things to us when we think positively, if you remember how connected the world is. At subatomic level, we are all just vast conglomerations of energy moving in a vast ocean of energy.

The more that I focus on what I do each day, rather than how I feel, the better I feel. By focusing instead on how I feel, and steering the day carefully around any delicate condition, I embrace not life but on this shortcoming that is interfering with my life. The key form of shortcoming that has blighted my life for 16 years is my tension headaches. I generally wake up with a headache. But now I 'just get on', and go about my daily tasks as best I can in spite of the headache. The more that I focus on those tasks, the less the headaches interfere. When I do not pay attention to them, they do indeed disappear – my brain tends to switch them off since I am not paying heed of them.

At the end of each day, when my focus has been on the activities within the day, rather than on how I felt, I go to bed with a more contented mind, and associations with headaches are reduced further. As I gain momentum in this lifestyle change, I am more and more likely to wake up just feeling good about life – *even if I have a headache* – since I know that it will barely affect my day.

6. Being more flexible

When I focus on what I want to do each day, I set out with the right intentions. But even the best intentions can be derailed off course. So I plan for the day with enough lightness that any changes of plan are easier to accommodate. I try to go with the flow. For someone with slight autistic tendencies, this is not so easy. I have an obsessional fondness for routine. This need for routine probably explains the large discomfort I tend to feel when my expectations are not met.

But the fact that being flexible is really not natural for me – that I am not genetically predisposed to go with the flow – does not mean that I cannot become more flexible. We are simply not told in school that with discipline, we can override our predispositions. I am training myself to be more flexible. It is tough and for me it is simply not instinctive. But each time I detect that my inflexibility is proving problematical, I flag it for attention. I do not – yet – have the instinct to be flexible, but I now have the instinct to spot when I am being inflexible and thereby start cultivating the flexible instinct.

7. Focusing more on people and events than material things

In my yearning for 'gadgets', I am very much a typical man. I also get caught up into thinking and believing that the next gadget that I am holding out to buy will raise my happiness level a notch. It is indeed likely to do so, but not the enduring elevation that I delude myself into thinking it will bring. Whilst I still indulge in gadgets and material things, I focus on the experiences they bring, and do not let them dominate my life. I try to avoid getting drawn into continually feeding my Apple iPad with new 'apps'. I bought it with the principle intention of playing and studying Oriental 'Go' games, and carrying out stock and share simulations. But it took only about 2 or 3 weeks for the novelty of the device to wear off. The urge to feed it new apps is the ego trying to seek the endless bursts of pleasure that it misguidedly believes will make me happy. With the novelty gone, I can focus on what I bought it for, rather than let it control me.

Likewise with people. If I go to the coffee shop to read but get embroiled in a conversation without a single word being read, then so be it. It is invariably more enjoyable than reading, and the book remains there to be read anyway another day. It has not gone away, and should not hold a grip on me. I try not to let material things govern me. Again, this is very much a work in progress.

Besides, people are ultimately what life is about. Leave the world exactly as it is and remove all the people, and all the material things in life would soon leave you feeling empty.

8. Accepting people without judging them

This is a particularly hard one to do, but I keep working at it. A few years ago when playing soccer, I used a silly name for a friend. He took offence and effectively ignored me for 2 or so years. I can talk with him now if I tread carefully. He is a great footballer, but prone to emotional intensity, and I evidently struck a nerve. But oh how easy it is to judge him for how he ostracised me. I do not harbour a grudge against him, not least for the obvious reasons that grudges are very damaging to health, eating away us from the inside long after their cause has gone. Much as my friend held a grudge against me for the silly name I called him.

But we do tend judge others on a regular basis. The more different someone is from us, the more intense our judgement. And this unfortunately reinforces social barriers, so I try hard to avoid this. But crucial to my ability in avoiding judgement is that I do not blame myself for instinctively judging in the first place. So I can kind of wipe the slate clean then, pushing away the instinct and treating the person as an equal, and try to see the world from their perspective. This is also a work in progress – I still find it very easy to see overtly arrogant people in a negative light, for example. The reality is that my dislike of arrogance is probably founded on slippery ground, and for sure, the strident confidence that such people has often allows them to get on in the world and achieve greatness.

9. Single tasking

Slightly off the beaten health track, but vital for my sanity, I have eventually learnt that when I have an intense single task to hyperfocus on, I perform much better than when I have to switch at irregular intervals between tasks. I tend to gain from the momentum of effort in one direction. Fragmented days, as I now call them, compromise my efforts, and are much more likely to bring my headaches to the fore.

So now, if I have two tasks to work on, rather than work on both each day, I dedicate alternate days to each. This suits how my mind works, and makes me happier and more productive.

10. Being honest with myself and others

For some strange reason, I find this an exciting habit. It often exhilarates me to be overtly honest with someone, especially about my own shortcomings. It relieves me of some of the burden of my weaknesses. By exposing them to others and to myself, and at the same time recognising that I never asked to have them in the first place disarms their power over me – their power to cause guilt or humiliation. But key here is not to revoke any responsibility for them. I still have to work at that.

I try to be honest with the motives behind my actions. I try to be honest with my feelings towards others. If I say I will do something, I do it.

11. Defusing the power of the ego

I have now established a reflex that kicks in when it detects my ego being greedy or intrusive. For example, when I bring a brand new ball to a game of soccer, my ego wants people to respect this. Now I try to just get on and play. When I knock something over and someone blurts out at how silly I was, my ego flares up seeking retribution for the hurt of their words. I now try to let the flare of defensive emotions fade. This has the long term effect of reducing their intensity over time, and of comments by others when they see that I do not 'bite'. I deal with the consequences of my clumsiness and then apologise if appropriate.

When my emotions carry me on a wave, I often fail to observe the ego's involvement. I might, for example, be having a friendly chat and find myself showing off about something, but only when it is too late. This is a hard aspect of the ego's grip to tackle. Striking a balance between spontaneous fun and employing vigilance to stop the ego hijacking the conversation to suit its ends is a hard, or maybe impossible one to achieve.

12. Not apologising for what I am

When I do something wrong, stupid or clumsy, like knocking something over, I apologise for my behaviour. My behaviour is the cause for my apology, not me as a person. I never choose to be clumsy! It is enough to have the problems that arise from clumsiness (in deed and in words) without further chastising myself for having been genetically endowed with this trait.

Basically, I accept what I am and do not defend it. But I do seek to limit damages where 'being me' causes problems. And I also tune into my environment to determine quite how much I can be myself.

13. Doing regular exercise

For those who know me, they may be surprised that I should need to *add* exercise to my weekly sporting regime. But the point of fact is that a wrist

223

injury for nearly 3 years has pretty well ruled out my regular tennis games, leaving me with soccer once or maybe twice a week. So I now make sure that 2 or 3 times a week, I walk 2 or 3 miles. It is surprisingly easy to get into this habit, but also very easy to slip out of it. Again, discipline is required.

14. Being happier

With repeated talk of discipline, it would appear that for me to he healthy is quite arduous. Yes, this is true. But I have a lot of bad habits that need realigning, and can already see huge benefits that are pretty well proportional to the efforts I have made so far.

But there is one aspect of health that I also look out for. I actively seek to be happy. Happiness also comes about naturally when I live according to what I am rather than how I feel, and when I work around problems, rather than let them defeat me. I also abide by the adage of not taking life or myself too seriously.

With all my newly invested habits bedding in, I now live life more lightly, and do simply laugh more. And when I laugh and it is maybe a little socially inappropriate, I care less. Better to laugh a bit too much than be sat dwelling on a headache.

15. Taking more risks

I try to do new and different things, and do not worry about making mistakes in the process. Better to embrace life than withdraw for fear of slipping up. Often, we are the only one judging ourself. No one told me to write this book. I am technically unqualified to write such a book, both in terms of my mastery (or not) of the English Language, and in my lay person understanding of the health matters I cover. But I did not let this stop me because I felt that I could offer enough in a holistic approach to health self help, allowing those with little time to read one book instead of dozens. I leave you to judge if this risk was a prudent one to take.

Appendix Two

Précis of this book

You have essentially finished the book. The intent of this chapter is to provide a future refresh of the ideas contained in the book. A distillation of the many and varied means to attaining good health.

Before I embark on this précis, it is wise to give one single summary of the message of the book. Good health is all about balance. It is no good eating impeccably if you take no exercise. It is not good for your health or the health of your family if you give them a bountiful life, but one bereft of your presence because you have to work excessive hours paying for it.

As I mentioned before, you do not have to adopt all ideas here to be healthy. It is generally enough to tackle the main areas in which you feel you have shortcomings in order to get back to a vibrant state of health. Health, after all, is more important than Wealth.

My suggestion is that you follow these basic guidelines :

- Adopt health improvements that will be of most value to yourself.
- Make these changes central to your life – apply them diligently, even if you are not used to doing this kind of thing.
- As you adopt them, recognise that change often moves you out of your comfort zone. Hang in there.
- Recognise that this change means you are not quite your 'normal self'. Do not let that this revert you to old habits.
- Others may start spotting changes in you, or maybe see that you are 'not your normal self', and want you to change back. Hang in there.

You must use determination to achieve change, and ignore the strangeness of the intermediate state.

- Changes will take as long as they have to. Hang in there.
- After a while, the benefits of the change will start to manifest themselves. This will reinforce the changes and make it easier to continue. But do not let this signal a desire to slacken off.

Many large towns and cities around the World today house fractured societies. Not only is the trend towards self sufficiency forcing the individual to be more important than the collective, but the loss of social cohesion is a perfect environment in which psychopaths can flourish. This 'sub-species' of human operate quite differently from the rest of us, principally characterised by a deficit of conscience. They can and do bludgeon their way through life with scant regard for the welfare of others, often reaching positions of power where they can wreak even greater havoc, driven as they are by their self serving nature.

As a means of raising the huge finances required for large scale projects such as the railways, the concept of corporations became firmly reestablished in the 19th Century. There was no theoretical limit to their funding, and many grew very large, and were subsequently able to provide the anonymity and power that psychopaths seek. It is no coincidence, therefore, that corporations exhibit psychopathic traits, but their impact goes well beyond the remit of any one psychopath in their employ. One consequence is that corporations regularly act in ways that are counter to the health and welfare of the public.

There are many methods used by big business to influence and manipulate the public, not least a coercion to become consumers of products that we did not even know we wanted. They use the media to promote their business needs ahead of our needs. They are often more powerful than governments, who they happily manipulate with financially-backed lobbying tactics. Ultimately, they have a callow and corrupting influence on our health. The pharmaceutical industry has subverted medicine into a money-making enterprise, relegating prevention and cure, the very fundamental basics of good health, to the sidelines. They do this in order to repeatedly 'treat' our symptoms with drugs that often do little more than introduce further symptoms via euphemistically named 'side-effects'. The very process of matching symptoms to drugs is of course flawed all along, failing as it does to take into account both the diversity of human biochemistry, and the diversity of the causes of any one symptom.

The pharmaceutical industry even have their tentacles inside the educational system, promoting drugs as the focus of medical treatment, and trivialising the effect of such important matters as nutrition and our minds on our health. The medical industry itself has grown too large, becoming more important than the patients it purportedly treats. Not only do they stick to this flawed symptom/drug approach to dealing with our health, but they also seek to take away our autonomy. We have been brain-washed into transferring our health management to 'authority'. An authority who happily push drugs onto us that can cause significantly greater damage to health than the illnesses they are alleged to remedy. The psychopathic pharmaceutical industry simply does not care, corrupted by the endless drive for profit and growth.

The equally psychopathic food industry is likewise driven to make profit at the expense of our health, bombarding us with aisle upon aisle of mass-produced foods that are laden with refined carbohydrates. They are even happy to manufacture food that is a by-product of industrial processes, disguising it in a palatable, but ultimately unhealthy form. The truth about our health is often hidden in simple and misleading messages from these big industries, and from governments. This is partly a result of the fundamental difficulty of communicating any information in a form that huge populations can comprehend. But a simple message often hides a very different reality. Even the scientific method, a key tool of industry, is often flawed in the very rigour that is supposed to be its prime asset. Yet it arrogantly dismisses anecdotal and empirical methods, even though these alternatives are legitimate in their own right, often yielding more meaningful and practical conclusions.

The scientific testing of drugs, intended as it is to protect the public, is often corrupted and subverted by the drug companies. But in spite of these malpractices, they do not have such an easy time in gaining drug approval because of a spanner in the works. The placebo effect. The mere act of being attended to, and administered a drug for our malady, even an inert sugar pill, can help improve our condition. Rather than explore and utilise the enormous power of belief that is the basis for the placebo effect, it is seen as an irritating factor that must be pushed aside in drug testing. The reality is that a part, and sometimes the whole part of the effect of a drug under test is itself the placebo effect. Medical training fails to recognise or capitalise on this influence of the mind on the body.

Many illnesses presented to doctors are not organic in nature, but caused by mind and emotion, even though they present real, physical symptoms. The influence of the mind on the body is perpetually trivialised. Self-fulfilling prophecies are a form of this influence, and can manifest themselves in strange ways. For example, the rapid decline in health of a man mistakenly diagnosed with terminal cancer. The same man who then made a fast and full recovery when informed of the mistake.

Since the 1950's, nutritional advice has been steered largely in the wrong direction, when Ancel Keys used flawed evidence to convince the US government that fat was bad for us. As soon as a direction is adopted by government, it is hard to budge them. The food industry used the fat-is-bad mantra to sell us grain-based products in preference to the labour intensive fat-laden animal products, reinforcing the fat-is-bad message. Subsequent research that clearly liberated fat from its guilty role was treated as anecdotal. Too much money was invested to change tack. Sadly, it was left to individuals to try to reinstate the importance of fat, especially the most-damned saturated fat, and the dangers of refined carbohydrates. Advisory bodies had been indoctrinated too long with the fat-is-bad mantra. So much so that they happily smeared Dr. Atkins when he introduced his low-carbohydrate diet, in spite of its success in helping millions of people safely and comfortably lose weight, many doing so effectively for the first time in their lives.

Most of our food starts from under our feet, yet the soil that the plants grown in that our animals eat is rarely treated with the importance that it deserves. Many soils have poor and unbalanced mineral levels, causing damage to plants, and the animals that eat them. Whilst this is a bad enough problem, the relentless drive by the food industry for faster, higher yields to satisfy their insatiable greed, results in an excessive use of chemicals. Nitrogen to boost plant growth, chemicals to protect the subsequent physically weakened state of fast growing plants, and chemicals to treat the animals who eat these chemical laden plants. The plant and animal food we eat is suffused with a cocktail of chemicals. And this chemical approach is actually so expensive (and hence counter productive), that farmers have to receive subsidies to be able to afford it. And the chemical industry is so happy with this boom in trade that they indirectly force almost all farmers to adopt this approach. Not content with vegetable, grain and meat product damage by chemicals, they also degrade our milk with pasteurisation and homogenisation processes.

Decades of research, by such visionaries as Weston Price, who travelled for ten years studying native diets, found that fat was very much innocent (and indeed vital to good health), and that it was these refined carbohydrates which were the guilty party. Guilty for causing many degenerative diseases. Most of those on traditional diets were free from tooth decay, and were blessed with wide jaws, free from tooth crowding. Yet the adoption of a Western diet, replete with refined carbohydrates resulted in narrow jaws within just one generation, along with higher incidences of mental retardation.

Low-calorie diets have been repeatedly shown to be ineffective in the long term, often causing weakness and a lowering in metabolism rather than weight loss. Low carbohydrate diets, high in fat have likewise been shown not only to be very effective but to be comfortable to follow. The apparent paradox that increased dietary fat results in lower bodily fat is sadly still denied by many, so strong is the fat-is-bad message. Yet fat is vital for many body parts and processes, and excess carbohydrates bad for the body, not least because they are prime fuel for cancer cells.

Big industry moved from fat to cholesterol as the big guilty food component, and managed to sell us statins, making billions each year in the process. Yet statins generally cause more damage than the high cholesterol they are meant to fix. The message that LDL cholesterol is bad for us is misguided – it is more the smallest LDL type that is indicted in heart disease – and this small type is more prevalent in diets rich in carbohydrates.

Most of us do not know that we have a second brain in our gut that controls our digestive system. It is called the enteric nervous system, and works in harmony with the brain in the heads of healthy people, via the vagus nerve. To maintain this harmony, we should eat slowly and in a relaxed state, for many with a food balance that favours fat ahead of carbohydrates. When carbohydrates are digested, insulin is released to marshal the resulting glucose from our blood stream to the cells of our bodies that need it, and to fat cells as a store for future energy. When excessive carbohydrates are consumed for long enough, cells can become resistant to the constant insulin coercion to accept glucose from the blood. This insulin resistance can lead to type 2 diabetes, and an eventual damage to the pancreas as it tires of releasing ever greater amounts of insulin in a hopeless struggle to lower the blood glucose levels. By adopting a low-carbohydrate diet, where fats become the larger source of energy, insulin levels are lowered, and the insulin resistance can gradually reverse. The higher fat levels in the diet additionally allow us to regulate food intake better, as the stomach is much better at sensing satiety via fat intake than carbohydrates, which leave the stomach rapidly. More sustained satiety and more stable blood sugar levels also create a much more stable state of mind, avoiding the mood swings that a high-carbohydrate diet can induce.

In the absence of low-carbohydrate diet endorsement by government or their advisory bodies, a plethora of self help books appeared. They spelt out the fat-is-good message via many different routes in order to differentiate themselves from other publications. There was justification in exploring different approaches for the simple reason that no one diet suits all. We have differing metabolisms, blood types, and life styles, and different diets were offered for variations such as these. For most, however, the simple avoidance of refined carbohydrates, and an acceptance of the health value of fat is a simple way to better nutritional health.

Physical exercise is a key component of a healthy lifestyle. It appears that regular exercise is best, and the more the better, injuries aside. Conversely, we cannot rest on our laurels – past exercise does not quite act as a future investment for our health as was initially believed. Use it or lose it, basically. Intense exercise not only releases endorphins, but also creates new brain cells in a part of the brain that is involved in receptivity to new experiences – making you engage in the World more. Exercise is therefore vital for the depressed, enabling them to re-engage with the World. Load bearing exercises are not just good for strong muscles, but also for strong bones, vital for the elderly. Static exercises such as yoga have more subtle effects, reducing compression on internal organs, and improving our breathing.

Alas, exercise can be compromised by injury. Just as with illness, this not only denies us the benefits of exercise as we recuperate, but can also cause a cascade of problems, not least isolating us from the main flow of life. Focusing on life rather than your ailment is a key to a healthy recovery.

Stress is of course a large factor in many illnesses, but it comes in two guises. Negative stress tears us apart, as we are literally pushed or pulled in two or more directions. Positive stress can be beneficial, however, allowing us to achieve more, as we work in a uniform, albeit tiring, direction. This is especially true for depressives who frequently underestimate their capacity to do things. They tire quickly, but if they keep pushing themselves – applying positive stress – they extend their capabilities.

But when any of us tire, we often do not know how to relax. We mistakenly believe that sat in front of the TV is relaxing, when in fact it is more engaging than calming. Better to learn to meditate, where you calm your mind by disengaging from the constant stream of subconscious chatter. Whilst banned as a dangerous drug, marijuana is also extremely good for relaxation and many other ailments. And so is melatonin, the hormone secreted by the pineal gland that controls our sleep patterns. When we age, melatonin levels drop, so we often wake before we are fully rested. Taking melatonin supplements can not only remedy this, but additionally enhances our immune system and possibly even extends our life.

Meaning in life is crucial to good health. It can of course come from work, but an excessive focus on your job can have a deleterious effect on your health. Having a diversity of life activities, including hobbies and maybe religious beliefs can protect us from the damaging effects of a loss in any one area of our lives. We are advised against putting all our eggs in one basket. Friends and family are key to our health – loneliness is actually measurably damaging to physical and mental health. But even when we get a good balance between work and play, and appear to have everything sorted, we can still be unhappy. Some people are driven to want more, in a never ending state of discontent at their lot. Many confuse pleasure with happiness, yet the former is transient, and the latter more the consequence of attitude than of material things or events. Research on happiness surprisingly reveals that very happy people actually make a point of being happy – they approach life with a focus on enjoying it regardless of what fate brings. They live in the moment, and avoid attachments – better to enjoy the fun of a gadget, but if you let it control you, any damage to the gadget becomes damage to yourself. Most governments focus on the economy, in the false belief that wealth equates with happiness. But it rarely does. Bhutan actually put the happiness of their people as their number one priority.

Many causes of unhappiness, and of mental and emotional suffering, are buried in our subconscious in the form of learned habits or 'schemas'. We might learn many 'shoulds' and 'musts' from our parents, not realising that they are like a straight jacket on our health. We can indeed change our habits – the brain is more flexible and adaptive than many realised until recent research showed otherwise – but to change requires mental discipline and determination. Yet we receive very little education for the need for such, and can rarely sustain the effort required to change. This is also largely due to the clinging nature of habits, and the unfamiliarity of both the change we are trying to adopt, and the difference in how we feel as we implement the change. So we easily find ways to abandon change, even though the benefits generally justify the effort.

The relentless stream of chatter from our subconscious mind tries to guide our behaviour, but it can also be over critical of us. Pathologically so, resulting in chronically low self-esteem in some people. We are not taught to value and love ourselves, and many problems stem from such an uncaring attitude to ourselves. We can also compound low self-esteem by treating each of our failures as defining us. By holding a more holistic, long term view of ourselves, we are no longer overtly affected by mistakes me make. We get a better balance. Many failures we make, and often repeatedly, stem from the wrong kind of thinking. Cognitive Behaviour Therapy addresses these habits, realigning thought processes, and thereby correcting our behaviours. Instead of focusing only on a double bogey in our round of golf, we turn our attention to the whole in two we got earlier. CBT corrects the kind of thinking that makes us see a date that goes badly wrong as meaning that we will never get a girlfriend again. When you start correcting bad habits like these, life flows better and your health improves radically.

Problems that arise from the wrong kind of thinking are not as drastic as those that arise from damaged emotions, in particular chronic anxiety. Anxiety is an expression of fear, and we are better off facing the fear rather than ignoring it, as the anxiety wants us to. But we must expect to feel the fear when we face it. It is just that each time we subsequently face the fear, it will reduce in its magnitude. Unfortunately, chronic anxiety can lead to panic attacks, a weak name for an extremely frightening state of fear that is often so intense that it feels as if we are about to die. Just as with general fear, we can tackle panic attacks by facing them, and then, paradoxically relaxing. But we must not read anything into the attack symptoms when we observe them, or we will release adrenaline and cortisone and exacerbate them. You cannot control them – you must let them fade in their own time.

This is true also of much of life. The more we try to control the World, the more frustrating life will be. By accepting whatever happens to and around us – by being aligned with reality – we can paradoxically handle it better. By trying to change the unchangeable, we merely stress ourselves. By expecting things to change, we put our life on hold until the changes happen. We are best accepting life now, change what we can, leave alone what we cannot, and not worry or concern ourself that we cannot get our own way all the time! Learn to "go with the flow", even if this is not in your nature.

Accept also that you have a dark side. Again, do not push away the reality that anger, jealousy, disgust and many other 'negative' emotions are part of you. But also recognise that you never asked for these – they are a part of your genetic inheritance – so do no punish yourself for having these emotions. And do not suppress them either – instead try to use reason to calm them down. Living in the thinking mind is likely to be much healthier for you than being caught up in an emotion controlled life.

One big driver of emotions is your ego. It makes you feel restless, endlessly driving you to acquire assets and status, and to be jealous of what others have. If you can release the grip of the ego, you can become more relaxed rather than driven, no longer coerced to buy things that you really don't need, or to dress simply to keep up with the latest fashions, driven in turn by an industry that keeps changing fashion simply to keep making money.

Try to be honest with yourself and others. And this means not only that you say what you mean, but that you do what you say you will. To treat others fairly, and with compassion and kindness, especially your offspring – a compassionate upbringing establishes a more healthy, relaxed baby and child, and this effect lasts throughout their life. But also, be compassionate to yourself – give yourself time to recover from overload, to rest, and thereby retain good health. This may sound selfish, but by ensuring you are healthy, you are then better positioned to help others.

References

AI	"Anatomy of an illness"	*****
	Norman Cousins, 2005	ISBN 978 - 0393326840

A uplifting example of recovery from life threatening illness. But it is rather more than that. Cousins demonstrated an ability to see beyond the dogma surrounding conventional treatment, swiftly transplanting himself from a grim hospital ward to a hotel room where he sat for days on end laughing at comedy videos.

Of course, the medical profession deemed him subject to spontaneous healing, dismissing his unusual approach as incidental. They kept their heads in their hands, not the slightest bit interested in pursuing any one-off recovery that failed to follow their rules.

AT	"Dr Atkins' New Diet Revolution : The no-hunger, luxurious weight loss plan that really works!"	****
	Dr. R. Atkins, 2003	ISBN 978 - 0091889487

The first Atkins book was a pivotal one in the history of nutrition for the masses. This was a wise, but somewhat late follow up. Alas, having discovered the efficacy of a low-carbohydrate diet with his own patients, and realised that the fat-is-bad message was a false dogma, his original book was too lax and ranting in style to be taken seriously by the medical profession.

This major rewrite starts in a similar vein, like a sales pitch. Fortunately, his tone totally changes when he covers the history and biochemistry of a low-carbohydrate diet. It is very much worth reading, but do so without tempering your view with the label that was applied to Atkins, and his diet, by the Medical profession. In essence, their defensive stance against him was probably more a reaction against his attack on their dogma than on the validity or otherwise of his diet.

Book ratings are entirely my own judgement :

***** Must read   **** Excellent   *** Good   ** Fair   * Poor

BC   **"The Body Code : 4 Genetic Types, 4 Diet Solutions"**   *****

Jay Cooper M.S., 2001   **ISBN 978 - 0671026202**

This book relies heavily on conjecture, with only a smattering of fact used as a guide. He takes the established body shape types (soma typing), glandular types, and (Ayurvedic) energy types, and synthesises 4 basic types of human. His synthesis is based on guesses at successful human psyches back to stone age times. From my perspective, he does not substantiate these properly. And he makes glib statements such as :

"The biochemical differences between humans begin with the reality that each of us has a unique set of ancestors, going back tens of thousands of years"

Well, I am one of 4 children, and we all shared the same parents and hence identical ancestors, yet we are vastly different in many ways.

He goes on to provide very detailed diets for each body type, but does so with zero explanation. The body code idea may have some merit, but not as presented here.

BI   **"Biochemical Individuality : The basis for the**   ********
genotrophic concept"

Roger Williams, B1 Ph.D, 1998   **ISBN 978 - 0879838935**

We are somewhat aware of how much humans vary in physical form and behaviour. But do we ever think about how we might differ internally. Mostly not – what we cannot se we tend to ignore.

This intriguing book reveals a similar, and sometimes greater diversity in the shape and biochemistry of our internals to our externals. It makes for a surprising read.

Did you know that the shape of heart valves, and hence their operation can vary significantly?

BR "The brain that changes itself" *****

Norman Doidge, 2008   ISBN 978 - 0131038872

Subtitled 'Stories of personal triumph from the frontiers of brain science', this is a fabulous, captivating read. Until recent years, it was strongly believed that the brain was no longer malleable beyond childhood. This was proven to be very wrong, as it was realised that the brain is very adaptive, or neuroplastic, and this is the core message of this book.

The underlying message is that we do not have to feel that limitations in our mental capacities or habits are fixed. The brain has evolved to evolve – to adapt to the World it encounters, and the range of ways it can adapt give confidence that you can improve your mind. Indeed, they established a number of programmes to achieve this, with profound effects on dyslexic and autistic children. Highly recommended, uplifting reading.

CM "The Compassionate Mind" ***

Paul Gilbert, 2009   ISBN 978 - 1849010986

Running to over 500 pages, this is not an easy read. It starts promisingly, and very enticingly, but slips into a rather more rambling style after the first hundred or so pages.

However, it is hard to criticise what is being said, even if it is hard to digest. It covers compassion and kindness from many angles, including of course the often ill practiced self compassion that is the starting point for our compassion for others.

CO "The Corporation : The pathological pursuit of profit ****
and power"

Joel Bakan, 2005   ISBN 978 - 1845291747

When first released on a mostly unknowing audience, this book caused a big stir. Coupled with a documentary movie by the same name, it brought to the surface a long overdue exposure of the practices and malpractices of corporations, the monolithic components of capitalism. Most unexpected, at least for myself, was that the legally defined nature of corporations *obliged* them to undertake undesirable behaviour if it best suited the interests of their shareholders.

DD "The Diet Delusion" *****

Gary Taubes, 2009   ISBN 978 - 0091924287

Published in the US as "Good calories, bad calories", this is the most authoritative book I have read on nutrition. In essence, it is more a history of nutritional science, along with the misguided nature of governmental nutritional advice. Taubes, a Science author, spent no less than 5 years researching and writing this book, interviewing 600+ specialists along the way. His obsession with detail appears to have left no stone unturned, but makes for a somewhat laboured read. I was running at about 20 pages an hour on a good day.

But the effort will reward you, as he goes to great depths to explain food metabolism, and how we have consistently been misinformed. His description of the cholesterol and triglyceride transport mechanisms, exposing the bad cholesterol myth is worth the price of the book on its own.

It should be mandatory reading for all government nutritional guidance agencies.

DI "Dr Bernstein's Diabetes solution" *****

Dr Bernstein, M.D., 2007   ISBN 978 - 0316167161

This appears to be a standard reference book for both type 1 and 2 Diabetes. The author was in his 70's at the time of writing, and in unusually robust health for someone who had suffered type 1 diabetes since aged 12.

He details the physiology of these conditions, and degenerative diseases that can result from them, many of which he suffered with in the 20 years his condition was mishandled.

He explains that he fine tuned his diet and insulin injections to achieve a stable blood sugar for the first time in 2 decades. A stability he sustained ever since. Required reading for all diabetics.

DP "The disease to please : curing the
people-pleasing syndrome"   *****

Harriet Braiker, Ph.D., 2002   ISBN 978 - 0071385640

For one who very much suffers the urge to please others, this
book reveals why I and others do this, often unaware of our own
ulterior motives. We are also often so frightened to break this
habit that we rarely do, frequently helping others begrudgingly
rather than willingly.

Via useful anecdote, this book helps understand the paradox that
saying no when appropriate helps us help ourselves, which allows
us to help others better.

EB "Evolve your brain"   *****

Joe Dispenza, D.C., 2007   ISBN 978 - 0757307655

Another overly long, but very valuable book. Joe's twin
understanding of brain biochemistry and behavioural psychology
allows him to explore and explain neuro-plasticity.

He aims to supply practical advice for radical reform of your own
mental health, even if you are currently already relatively
healthy. Alas, his long winded style does serve to water down and
confuse his messages, but the book is still worth 5 stars because
of the value of his ideas.

EC **"The Emotion Code"** ***

Dr. Bradley Nelson, 2007 **ISBN 978 - 0979553707**

The epitome of a concept developed empirically and expounded by anecdote. Nelson uses an effortlessly easy style of writing to convey somewhat esoteric material. At times, however, he lost me completely in his bold declarations of exactly how the body holds onto the energies of emotion. What he describes can neither be measured nor observed, so his confidence is disconcerting. The remit of the book is to explain the emotional storage mechanism and to supply a number of ways to determine and release your own particular trapped emotions. At the time of writing, I have not tried any, but if his anecdotes are to be believed, the effect of release can be as profound as it is rapid. I look forward to trying.

EG **"Evil Genes: Why Rome fell, Hitler rose, Enron failed** ****
and my sister stole my Mother's boyfriend"

Barbara Oakley, 2008 **ISBN 978 - 1591026655**

A good discussion of the nature of psychopathy, illustrated with meaningful examples. She also theorises on the likely causes of the prevalence and survival of this anti-social trait.

EN **"The Emperor's new drugs : exploding the anti-** *****
depressant myth"

Professor Irving Kirsch, 2009 **ISBN 978 - 1847920836**

Do not be deterred by the brevity of this book, where the main narrative runs to much less than 200 pages. It is an authoritative recounting of placebo research that dug so deep that it unveiled not only widespread corruption of drug trial results, but involvement of the FDA in denying the public the truth about drugs.

But the most telling conclusion of this timely book is that the efficacy anti-depressant drugs is simply down to a super placebo effect. And this 'super' effect is simply supplied by the side effects! The bigger the side effect, the more effective the anti-depressant effect. Enlightening but very worrying that billions appear to have been made from super placebo pills.

ER "Eat right 4 your type" **

Dr P. J.D'Adamo + C. Whitney, 1998   ISBN 978-0712677165

The first in a series of books (see "Live right 4 your type") that place great importance of your blood type on your biochemistry and physiology and hence create a need to eat accordingly. They claim to back up their recommendations with many successful clients/patients.

The idea appears to have merit, but no explanation is given for the detailed diets, and I smell a rat here. They state, for example, that Blood type A should not eat pork. Nor should blood type B, or O or AB. Quite what their logic or agenda is I cannot fathom.

FE "Flat Earth News" ****

Nick Davies, 2009   ISBN 978 - 0099512684

Subtitled "An award-winning reporter exposes falsehood, distortion and propaganda in the global media", this is a long overdue exposure of an accelerating destruction of quality, factual, impartial news reporting. At least as much as that has ever been possible.

As a newspaper journalist for some decades, Davies covers the original, long standing good practices, and how they have been increasingly eroded in the ruthless drive to cut costs and increase profits, leaving the door open for misinformation. The book does drag somewhat, in my opinion, but is otherwise a good read.

FF "Feel the fear and do it anyway" *****

Susan Jeffers, 2007   ISBN 978 - 0091907075

Probably the de-facto popular book for countering your fears. Well written, but sometimes a little optimistic in its outlook, it describes the counter intuitive approach to handling various types of fear. These fears tend to affect pretty well all of use at one time or other in life. The key concept is to avoid running from the fear, and live through the experience. The theory is that we often expect greater fear than actually transpires, and that having survived, we are likely to tone down the fear response the next time.

FG "Feeling Good : The new mood therapy" ****
David B. Burns   ISBN 978 -D30380810338

The first mass market book about CBT (Cognitive Behaviour Therapy), written by one of the CBT founders. Overly long and detailed as a primer, but it can be treated as such by reading just the first 100 or so pages, and learn a great deal both about yourself, and your habits, and how to break or temper them.

It compares the efficacy of CBT in relation to medication, and then proceeds to detail the cognitive distortions that underlie mental and social health difficulties. Do not underestimate how pervasive these are – I ticked all the boxes for the wrong kind of thinking.

FI "Food Inc.: A participant guide" ***
Karl Weber   ISBN 978 - 1586486945

Ambitiously subtitled : "How Industrial food is making is sicker, fatter, and poorer and what you can do about it", the book starts with some splendid and insightful writing, but sadly deteriorates afterwards. It is a collection of essays to accompany the documentary film by the same name. Alas, for many writers, it appears to be a platform for shouting about very narrow areas of concern that do not particularly concern you and I directly enough.

FP "Food Politics : How the food industry influences **** nutrition and health"
Marion Nestle   ISBN 978 - 0520254039

Complete with 3 awards, I was really looking forward to reading this book. It appears to have a great sense of authority, but, to my view, is flawed by dogma. As an ex Government nutrition adviser, Nestle was so steeped in the traditional dogma on good food health (re fat is bad, saturated fat is extra bad), that her motives are undermined by a lack of enlightenment. It Is difficult to read the vast amount of detail she offers when she can glibly state that "The cause if overweight is an excess of calories consumed over calories burned off in activity". But it easily deserves 4 stars because it exposes the power the food industry has to heavily influence the nutritional advice to the masses.

GL "The Glycemic Load Diet" **

Rob Thompson, 2006   ISBN 978 - 0071462693

Yet another diet book, seeking to carve out another niche. But ultimately flawed – the glycemic index is a relatively crude guide to the speed and nature with which we metabolise food. Basing a diet book on just this aspect of nutrition alone is too limited.

GR "Gut reaction" ****

Gudrun Jonsson, 1998   ISBN 978 - 0091816735

A splendid, enlightening little book, elevating the importance of our much disregarded digestive system. And introducing the enteric nervous system – the 'brain' in our guts that controls much of our digestive processes. As you will learn, 'gut feeling' has a physiological legitimacy.

HH "How we choose to be happy" ****

Rick Foster and Greg Hicks, 2004   ISBN 978 - 0399529900

The subtitle "The 9 choices of extremely happy people - their secrets, their stories" pretty well summarises the book. The authors toured the World studying the attributes of people identified by locals as supremely happy.

The conclusions are not entirely obvious, and it is questionable if you could mimic them in the long term, or indeed whether these 'choices' are the cause or consequence of a chirpy outlook.

HM "How your mind affects your body" ****

David R. Hamilton PhD., 2008   ISBN 978 - 1848500235

A well coordinated array of mid-body aspects are covered here, with particular attention paid to recent research into the placebo effect. It rightly points out that the often marginalised placebo effect is now taking centre stage.

The book would have received 5 stars if Hamilton had added more of his own ideas rather than 'merely' collating material from his researches. But, such material is of high value, so all is not lost.

HS **"The Highly Sensitive Person : How to survive and** ***
thrive when the World overwhelms you"

Elaine N. Aron, 1999   ISBN 978 - 0272253968

A great concept, and reasonably well executed. I am not entirely convinced with the precise and large figure of 20% given for the number of highly sensitive people in the population. Nor how the same percentage can be proven to apply across the animal kingdom. But nevertheless it is good to read that you are neither as extreme as you thought, and that by being at one end of a spectrum, you can give yourself more slack than you probably are.

HU **"Human evolution : An illustrated introduction"** ****

Roger Lewin, 2004   ISBN 978 - 1405103787

A good primer on evolution for students, with excellent illustrations as the title might suggest. It enlightened me with regard the speed of evolutionary change.

HY **"Hypoglycemia : The classic handbook completely** ***
revised and updated"

J. Saunders, Dr. Harvey M. Ross, 2002 ISBN 978 - 0758201324

Hypoglycaemia is a slightly controversial 'condition', often rejected as a possible ongoing problem by the medical profession. They see it only as a possible diabetic state. The author has every right to think differently as she lost her daughter as a result of the condition, and advocates a greater respect for it.

She covers the difficulties of diagnosis, consequences and then essentially covers life style changes and foods to avoid.

JM	"Junk Medicine : Doctors, lies and the addiction bureaucracy"	*****
	Theodore Dalrymple, 2007	ISBN 978 - 1905641598

A highly controversial topic handled with eloquence. He argues very persuasively that the 'war on drugs' is a political self fabrication that has become a self sustaining beast – as all the players act out the war in a self fulfilling prophecy of titanic scale.

Read it and get a more enlightened picture.

KD	"The Ketogenic Diet: A complete guide for the Dieter & the practitioner"	****
	Lyle McDonald and Elzu Volk, 2000	ISBN 978 - 0967145600

Unlike many mass market books on health or nutrition, the authors have no axe to grind – this is an impartial look at diets that are low enough to trigger the ketogenic state. It is also a very detailed, knowledgeable exploration of the subject, and appears to be the de facto reference book on the subject.

Unlike most low-carb books, it intelligently covers intensive exercise, and the value of temporarily boosting carbohydrate intake to sustain the high bodily demands. It would have received 5 stars if it had not become too technical and intense. You may value it well because it does *not* tread so lightly.

IR	"Irrationality"	*****
	Stuart Sutherland, 2007	ISBN 978-1905177073

Not many people are terribly aware that their minds regularly delude them. It is not so much that delusional, irrational behaviour is universal, but how many areas of our life it affects. Backed by copious research, this superb book is a chilling expose of the blinkered nature of our conscious mind.

Highly recommended for those who want to be self aware. Frightening for those who do not.

IS "Infinite Self : 33 Steps to Reclaiming Your Inner *****
Power"

Stuart Wilde, 1996   ISBN 978 - 1561703494

Just over 200 pages of mostly brilliant, succinct writing about
Taoism, the Oriental philosophy. The essence of the writing is the
recommendation to move away from an ego driven life to one
that stems from an internal energy that is itself part of the life
force connecting all things.

Whilst this sounds ethereal, it rapidly becomes sensible. Taoism
aside, this book is chock full of nuggets of wisdom. Much of the
writing makes for effortless reading, but at the same time,
profound in its meaning.

LM "Limits to Medicine : Medical nemesis - the ****
expropriation of health"

Ivan Illich, 2001   ISBN 978 - 1842300077

One of those writers who can slip between the most elegant and
the most turgid of prose. But there is enough of the former to
make this an insightful read. His thinking penetrates through the
ordinary, seeing it for what it is and what it could be.

The book focuses on latrogenesis – namely the generation of ill
health by Physicians. It is a legitimate claim, one that he flushes
out to endless depths, making you almost afraid of entering a
medical establishment again.

LR "Live right 4 your type" ****

Dr P. J.D'Adamo + C. Whitney, 2002   ISBN 978-0140297850

An extension of the theme of "Eat right 4 your type", it has been
debunked by a number of reviews. But lifestyle according to your
blood type is popular in Japan, where application forms even ask
you to declare your blood type. An attempt is made to lace the
writing with an air of authority with frequent references to a gene
for blood type that is linked with many other matters. I am
personally not convinced.

LW	"Loving what is : How four questions can change your life"	**
Byron Katie,2002		ISBN 978 - 0712629300

Following an epiphany, where she went into a deep and sustained state of acceptance, fighting against nothing at all in her life, loving all and everything around her, Katie has one of the clearest experiences of the concept of acceptance. Namely, to accept what is going on around you without the regular urges to reject or change things.

This book takes the concept to an extreme, however, matching the depth she was able to achieve. The consequence is that she misses the key counterpoint to the concept of acceptance – that it does not excuse you the responsibility of making change where appropriate. She tends to advocate a form of acceptance that is far too passive.

For example, she describes her son watching TV, catching her thought "he shouldn't be watching so much", and just accepting that this was simply what he did. Here, acceptance is too detached – it is correct to accept the reality of the situation, but not to let it stay that way.

The 4 key questions that form her acceptance philosophy probably do work well, but the sample narratives are irritatingly peppered with the word 'darling', undermining her messages.

ME "Melatonin"   *****

R. Reiter, Ph.D, J. Robinson, 2003   ISBN 978-0553574841

A colleague of mine could not believe that a book on a single hormone could run to 400 pages. The point here is that this is not just any old hormone. Well, it is in one sense – melatonin is probably the only hormone to remain totally unchanged across virtually all animals in 3 billion years or so. But it is a very special hormone, having broad effects on sleep, sex, aging and your immune system. Written by one of the early researchers, this is an authoritative tome. Read it and buy some.

MM "The mind made flesh : essays from   ****
the frontiers of psychology and
evolution"

Nicholas Humphrey, 2002   ISBN 978-0192802279

An insightful and diverse set of essays revolving around the human condition. It is here that I encountered the insightful and logical essay on the theory of the origin of the placebo effect.

But the book is worth reading beyond that chapter, his writing readily drawing you into his ideas and thinking.

MS "The Mask of Sanity"   ****

Hervey Cleckley M.D., 1941   ISBN 978-0452253411

This is the original definitive psychopathy reference. The nature of 1940's writing makes it a somewhat laboured read, but a deeply insightful one. Most revealing is the long series of case studies. Whilst you can sense a pattern of behaviour and personality type in these studies, it is hard to pin it down. This is in part because psychopathy is a spectrum disorder, so manifests to varying degrees, but also because the fundamental lack of conscience that characterises psychopathy interacts with personality in many rich and diverse ways.

He goes on to define the salient attributes of psychopathy, differentiating them from narcissism for example. A laboured but valuable read.

MT	"The Metabolic typing Diet"	***
	W. Wolcott and T. Fahey, 2002	ISBN 978-0767905640

Underlying this book is the sensible recognition that human diversity is enormous, and therefore that there can be no one diet that fits all. They claim that by addressing nutrition (and nutrition alone it seems), that the consequence will be a diminishing of ailments. This narrowness of view devalues the book in my view. Which is a shame as it covers some key concepts well, such as a well written undermining of the current medical simplistic symptom-drug habit.

ND	"Nutrition and physical degeneration"	****
	Weston A Price, DDS, 2008	ISBN 978-0916764203

As a highly regarded dentist in the early part of the 20th century, Price was frustrated at the lack of research into healthy teeth and jaws. He could not believe that only dental *problems* were ever researched. So he embarked on a 10 year travel around the World to investigate people eating traditional diets, and the effect it hand on their teeth.

His discovery of wide jaws with no teeth crowding, and extremely low levels of decay were profound. He was able to correlate dental and general health with a diet rich in quality vitamins and minerals and fat, and inversely correlate with refined foodstuffs. From Switzerland to Africa, the message was the same.

The high quality of health he found was also matched by a lack of degenerative diseases. He was able to mostly rule out genetic factors as an explanation since those natives who adopted a Western diet, rich in refined carbohydrates, invariably rapidly lost their good health. The writing is somewhat heavy going, otherwise it would have received 5 stars.

ON "Optimal Nutrition"   ***

Dr. Jan Kwaśniewski, 1999   ISBN 83 - 87534 - 13 - 7

Over a period of some 20 years, this Polish Physician fine tuned the diets of obese and ill patients in his charge. As a result of his efforts he determined a beneficial diet. He claims a scientific basis to the precise ratios of Protein to Fat to Carbohydrates in this diet that will result in optimal health. He covers some of the science, but the book in general is written with very poor discipline, erring on the side of a supreme optimism in his judgements.

However, there is no denying the weight of practical support for this diet, to the tune of 2 million Poles, and a few dozen doctors who recommend it. He claims that low carbohydrate, adequate protein and masses of fat in the diet will clear long standing conditions, even liberating type 1 diabetics from insulin injections. I feel, however, that he undermines this huge weight of anecdotal support by failing to cover the diet logistics with enough authority. But this is an important book nevertheless. It appears that the book can currently only be obtained by mail order from Poland. This is at least how I got my copy.

PA "Physical Activity : and Health"   ***

A. E. Hardman, D. J. Stensel, 2009   ISBN 978 - 0415421980

This elegantly produced textbook on the effect of exercise on health was somewhat disappointing. It was extremely thorough in its coverage of research method and stats, but the weight of such information left little room for useful facts – any tangible benefits of physical activity on health.

PL "Placebo : Mind over matter in modern medicine"   ***

Dylan Evans, 2004   ISBN 978 - 0007126132

Whilst a great book concept, I felt that he lost the good pace of early chapters and became engrossed in a complex analysis and theory of the operation of the placebo effect. There are probably more accessible books on this subject.

PM "The Plastic Mind"   ★★★★
Sharon Begley, 2009   ISBN 978 - 1845296742

Close to the cutting edge of the very recent field of neuroplasticity, this is an interesting book that also looks at the effect of Buddhist meditation on the brain and mind. But at its core, it investigates the originally taboo concept that the mind can change the brain – that thinking can manifest as physical neuronal change.

This was nowhere more evident and demonstrable than in monks who bravely sat in fMRI scanners. Especially those who practiced compassionate meditation. A lively, gripping book.

PP "The Protein Power Lifeplan"   ★★
M. R. Eades and M. Dan Eades, 2001   ISBN 978 - 0446678674

The title of this book misleads. It principally promotes the low-carbohydrate diet advocated by Atkins and Groves etc. That aside, this mighty tomb goes into great depth on a whole array of nutritional health matters, from the truth about cholesterol to the danger of high/low carbohydrates. And therein lies a weakness, in my view. It goes to deep, and becomes a general health guide, losing focus, and often the readers attention. But it is still an authoritative book on nutritional health, and worth reading.

S1 "The Schwarzbein Principle : The truth about losing   ★★★★
weight, being healthy and feeling younger"
Diana Schwarzbein, M.D., 1999   ISBN 978 - 1558746800

S2 "The Schwarzbein Principle II : A regeneration process   ★★★★
to prevent and reverse accelerated aging"
Diana Schwarzbein, M.D., 2002   ISBN 978 - 1558749641

The first 2 books in a series that take a more balanced and holistic approach to low-carbohydrate eating. You should eat the *right* amount of carbs, so as to avoid hormonal imbalances. The hormonal concept is extended to cover all life aspects. The concern I have about these books is that they appear to fall into the common trap of milking a good idea too far, extrapolating without quite enough convincing evidence, especially with regard the reversing of aging. Otherwise, the books are highly recommended.

SD "How to stop your doctor killing you" ***
Vernon Coleman, 2003 ISBN 978 - 1898947141

Coleman is an amazingly prolific author, writing with great passion and seemingly great knowledge about diverse matters. Here, he lays into Doctors, and, it seems, for very good reason. However, whilst there is a lot of common sense in this book, it is in essence a rambling rant, without enough care and attention taken to organise the contents. Or to qualify statements with references.

SE "Self Esteem : A proven program of cognitive ****
techniques for assessing, improving and maintaining
your self-esteem"
M. McKay, Ph.D + P. Fanning ISBN 978 - 1572241985

A thorough analysis of the causes of self esteem, and detailed, but time consuming techniques for getting it back on track. My own feeling is that the methods are very involved, and therefore require a lot of diligence to stick to. Certainly, whilst reading the book will help in itself, without taking the exercises on board, you would appear to miss the main message from the book.

SH "Self help for your nerves : Learn to relax and enjoy *****
life again by overcoming stress and fear"
Claire Weeks, 1995 ISBN 978 - 0722531556

This slim book is a life saver. A brilliantly incisive, effective and reassuring guide to overcoming both panic attacks and the slide into a nervous breakdown. The authority with which she writes allows you to accept as legitimate the claim that no matter how far you are in decline towards a fully fledged nervous breakdown, you can arrest and reverse it.

I lent a copy of this book to my Doctor, who now refers it to panic attack sufferers. It helps you understand how your anxiety manifests in alarming symptoms that are aggravated by your instinct to worry about them. She helps you break this cycle. Most sufferers fail to do this because the method is slightly counter intuitive.

SI "Sick and tired of feeling sick and tired" ****

P. J. Donoghue, Ph.D, M. E. Siegel, ISBN 978 - 0393320657
Ph.D, 2000

An eminently sensible and practical book, subtitled "Living with invisible chronic illness", it differentiates between organic and functional illnesses. The latter can be just as physically debilitating, but are, it is explained, of emotional and/or cognitive origin. The book covers such causes and the remedial action that can be taken. An enlightening read.

SL "The Spirit Level" ****

Richard Wilkinson & Kate Pickett ISBN 978 - 141032368

A thorough, but mostly unsettling account of the inverse relation between the degree of income disparity in a country and the health and happiness of its people.

SP "Spark : The effect of exercise on the brain" *****

John Ratey & Eric Hagerman, 2009 ISBN 978 - 1847247209

A hugely entertaining and uplifting book, as long as you happily embrace exercise in the first place. If you do not, you may wince at the benefits that accrue from exercise, the more intense, regular, and life long the better. Whilst the book moves from easy reading chapters of an anecdotal nature, to overly technical discussions of brain operation, it is still a worthy 5 star read.

SS "Snakes in suits : When Psychopaths go to work" ****

P. Badiak, Ph.D, R. Hare, Ph.D, 2007 ISBN 978 - 0061147890

You many not like what you read, especially if you have personal involvement of the ruthless charm of fast rising psychopaths at your place of work. The book covers the types of work-environments psychopaths flourish in and the techniques they use to flourish. Frightening reading, as you learn about humans who act as if they were a predatory, parasitic or scavenging animal. Yet, they mostly go undetected – when the whistle does blow, they have recruited enough higher Management support to devalue the whistle blower's message. And once that happens, no one dares try again, leaving the way open for them to rise to the top. Scary stuff I am afraid.

RA	"Radical Acceptance : embracing your life with the heart of a buddha"	****
	Tara Brach, Ph.D., 2004	ISBN 978 - 0553380996

An enlightening read, explaining how we get subverted by both our ego and the way in which society manipulates our ego. Suffering is a part of life and we should accept it - hence the radical nature of this book on acceptance.

TM	"Take me to truth : Undoing the ego"	***
	Nouk Sanchez, Tomas Vieria, 2007	ISBN 978 - 1846940508

A competent book covering the release of control that the ego can have on your life. I was less than convinced by the organisation of this release into six stages – it was not always clear what each stage was trying to achieve (unlike the supreme clarity in no less than 33 stages in "Infinite Self").

TT	"Trick and Treat"	*****
	Barry Groves, 2008	ISBN 978 - 1905140220

The result of 26 years of full time, independent research into nutrition and health. Groves had adopted a low-carb/high-fat diet since 1962, yet was perpetually ridiculed by colleagues. Yet he was extremely healthy on the diet, so he was highly motivated to explore the truth of the matter, especially as it was seen as directly opposed to 'rational', recommended nutritional advice. The book does repeat itself, and makes digressions to discuss matters such as sunshine, but it has a lot of important messages to impart.

It has had a greater influence on me than any other non-fiction book I have read. It is easy to describe books as profound and life changing, but this one performed these roles effortlessly.

The title refers to the *trick* employed by the food and pharmaceutical industries to make us ill, allowing them to then *treat* us for those ailments.

US "Use of the self" ★★★★
F. M. Alexander, 1985   ISBN 978 - 0575037205

A great little book, taking you into the life of an extraordinarily patient and perceptive man. Who else would have been able to determine that his posture was the cause of a sore throat by observing himself act in front of mirrors for months!

The book is largely an academic discussion, not intended as a practical guide. But accepting this limitation, it is very enlightening beyond posture, revealing quite how stubborn our ingrained habits are. Who has tried to change their tennis stroke, only to swiftly revert back to their old ways, even though it has consistently failed them, simply because it is where our comfort zone is. Change takes us away from our comfort zone. You would be advised to get an illustrated book on the Alexander Technique if you want to learn and apply his ideas.

WC "Without Conscience : The disturbing World of the Psychopath among us" ★★★★
Robert D. Hare, Ph.D, 1999   ISBN 978 - 1572304512

The classic modern book on Psychopathy. A much simpler and more accessible, but lighter equivalent to "The mask of sanity". He adds his own explanations for the continued prevalence of this 'sub-class' of humans. A good general primer on the subject.

WH "Wheel of health : The sources of long life and health among the Hunza" ★★★
G. T. Wrench, 2006   ISBN 978 - 0486451541

Originally written in 1938, the author visited the Hunza people in Northern Pakistan, and describes their good health and the nutrition behind it. A detailed example of life without refined foods.

WL "Weight loss for the mind" ★★★
Stuart Wilde, 2004   ISBN 978 - 1561705375

This is a neat pocket book on releasing the ego's grip on your life. But it is tiny and of use only, it appears, as a *portable* reminder of a healthy way of thinking and living.

WK "Why kindness is good for you" ***

David R. Hamilton PhD, 2010   ISBN 978 - 1848501782

A relatively short and simple book, but with quite a few interesting observations about the profound effect of kindness on ourselves and others.

WW "We want real food" *****

Graham Harvey, 2006   ISBN 978 - 1854292676

This book took me by surprise, exposing quite how little I (and presumably many others) knew about both the enormous importance and the structure of the soil beneath our feet. A large part of the surprise was that the minerals in the vegetables we cultivate and pick is principally sourced from rock dust in the soil. If the dust is depleted, or imbalanced, then the soil is damaged, the plants that grow in it suffer, the animals that eat it suffer, and we who eat the animals do likewise. A classic food chain problem that was new to me.

What is less surprising, but deeply sad, is that the current 'standard practice' of cultivating plants with boosting and regulating chemicals destroys the mineral content of the soil. And you can guess what happens to the food that grows there. It may look the part, but will be depleted and imbalanced in micronutrients. As well as be loaded with applied chemicals.

This is a very important book, and in spite of mundanity of the subject, and a fair bit of repetition, it is an easy, revelatory read. Highly recommended.

YE "Yellow on the outside : Asian culture on the inside" ****

Anson Chi, 2005

Available as a free ebook on the Internet, this is a fun, light read, written by an east Asian, about east Asian culture. It is a novel, and a repetitive one, but also an insightful one. In extreme summary, about how very much status drives so much of oriental culture, to the point where self sufficiency precludes the natural and health giving action of hugging each other. Even parents would rarely hug their children.

Index

A

A1 beta casein 74
A2 beta casein 74
acceptance   155, 165, 184, 186, 190, 193, 214
acupuncture 48
Adenosine Triphosphate (ATP) 89
ADHD - Attention deficit hyperactivity disorder 50
adrenaline 90, 118, 135, 157, 184
agendas 10
agriculture 78
alcohol 10, 27, 93, 132, 135
Alexander technique 154, 171
Alexander, F.M. 125, 151
Alpha-Linolenic Acid (ALA) 18
alternative medicine 48, 154
Alzheimer's disease 140
American Diabetic Association (ADA) 52
American Heart Association (AHA) 67
American Medical Association (AMA) 66
American Physiological Society (APS) 115
amygdala 171, 189, 214
Amylases 93
anaesthetics 48, 116, 121
anecdotal method 23, 35
anecdotal 20, 22, 60, 62
anger 123, 157, 165, 172, 178, 190, 191
anti-depressants 29, 30, 32, 50, 112, 115, 172
anti-oxidant 135
anxiety   90, 122, 123, 158, 180, 182, 183, 189, 200
apologising 169
Aron ,Elaine 180
aspartame 94
aspergers syndrome 72, 132, 181
aspirin 24, 134

atherosclerosis 64
Atkins diet 66, 103
Atkins, Dr. Robert 66, 104
Attention Deficit Hyperactivity Disorder (ADHD) 115, 130, 132
attention 115, 129, 182
Atwater, Wilbur 60
auditory cortex 121
autonomy 48
Avandia 51

B

Banting, William 60, 62, 66
Baum, Michael 149
Begley ,Sharon 211
Benedict, Francis, Gano 61
Bernstein, Dr. 99
Bextra 52
Bhutan 149
biochemistry 42, 43
blood sugar 9, 63, 87, 93, 95, 96, 99, 101, 185
blood type 106
Brach ,Tara 191
Braiker ,Harriet 162
breathing 117
Buddhism 121, 129, 211
Burns ,David 171
butter 55, 56, 81, 110

C

caffeine 27
calories 59, 61, 62, 76, 85, 86, 94, 101, 119
cancer 28, 35, 40, 79, 83, 87, 88, 89, 94, 109, 127, 131, 135, 149
cannabis 131
capitalism 148, 160, 200
carbohydrates 17, 44, 59, 60, 61, 62, 66, 67, 69, 79, 81, 82, 87, 89, 93,

95, 96, 98, 99, 101, 104, 105, 106, 107, 108, 109, 134
Cardiovascular Disease (CVD) 64
Cardiovascular Heart Disease (CHD) 116
cardiovascular-health 68
cars 147, 148
cattle 73, 76, 81
causal relationships 22
cerebellum 115
charity 213
cheese 81, 101
chemical industry 73
cholesterol 66, 67, 89, 90, 91
Chronic Fatigue Syndrome (CFS) 122
Cleckley, Hervey 3
Co-Enzyme Q10 89, 104
coconuts 63, 82
Cognitive Behaviour Therapy (CBT) 167, 171, 177, 204
comfort zone 155, 157, 183, 204, 205
community 212, 215
compassion 185, 201, 210, 213
complaining 196, 205
confrontation 165
Conjugated Linoleic Acid (CLA) 73
conscience 2, 3
consumerism 11, 12, 148, 199
contraindications 24
control 186
Cooper, Jay 105
core beliefs 162, 167, 177
corporations 4, 5, 6, 7, 9, 10, 12, 211
corruption 23
Cousins, Norman 20, 49
criticism 165, 195
cure 39

D

Dalai Lama 211
Dalrymple, Theodore 131
dark side 192

de novo glucogenesis 104
deflection 10
dementia 141
dentate gyrus 114
depression 22, 31, 33, 112, 114, 119, 120, 131, 136, 142, 167, 172
diabetes 51, 52, 60, 95, 98, 109, 136
    type 1 96, 99, 109
    type 2 44, 96, 97
diet 60, 61, 62, 63, 66, 67, 80, 81, 82, 84, 87, 95, 98, 99, 102, 105, 106, 107, 108
digestion 91, 92, 101, 214
discipline 144, 207
Dispenza ,Joe 155
diversity 17
doctors 26, 38, 42, 43, 45, 46, 48, 53, 67, 80, 90, 104
Dodds, Sir Charles 63
Dososahexaenoic Acid (DHA) 18, 73
drug research 50
drug testing 21, 23, 24, 25, 26, 28, 30, 31, 34, 51, 133
dyslexia 72, 158

E

economics 12
economy 11
ectomorphs 105
education 14, 45, 53, 55
Effexor 32
eggs 77, 88, 110
ego 198, 199, 205, 206, 210
Eicosapentaenoic Acid (EPA) 18, 73
elderly 36, 114, 134
electronic devices 146, 148
emotions 171, 177, 179, 182, 187, 189, 194, 196, 197, 205, 211, 214
empirical method 22, 24, 108
empirical 21
endomorphs 105
endorphins 114, 116, 118, 214

energy 201
enzymes 75, 92, 93
epigenome 84
epilepsy 98
exercise 22, 61, 96, 111, 118, 137, 172
expectations 37, 194, 198, 200, 202

F

fats 55, 56, 59, 60, 61, 62, 63, 64, 65, 66, 69, 74, 76, 85, 86, 87, 90, 93, 95, 98, 99, 105, 107, 108, 110
FDA 18, 51, 57
fear 122, 155, 179, 183, 195
fertilisers 72
fibre 67, 104
Fibromyalgia 122
fish 80, 82
flexibility 196, 197, 204
Food and Agriculture Organisation (FAO) 87
food industry 54, 55, 56, 63, 67, 72, 73, 74, 76, 148
Food Standards Agency (FDA) 68
Framington study 90
free fatty acids 87, 104
Freud, Sigmund 199
frontal cortex 130, 172, 177
frontal lobes 34
fruit 17, 55, 69, 80, 94
functional illness 122

G

gall bladder 93
generalisations 205
genetics 81, 84, 86, 142, 154, 164, 172, 177, 185, 191, 193, 199
Gilbert, Paul 164, 177
giving 144, 214
glycemic index 94, 106, 134
glyconutrients 57

governments 7, 9, 10, 13, 16, 17, 51, 53, 61, 65, 72, 106, 131
grains 55, 56, 68, 73, 78, 79, 101
grass 73
Groves, Barry 99

H

habits 152, 156, 162, 171, 179, 182
happiness 11, 12, 130, 142, 146, 149, 150, 160, 196, 197, 200, 202
headaches 80, 102, 120, 121, 122, 123, 129, 161, 167, 182, 188, 207
heart attacks 65
heart-disease 22, 60, 67, 82, 89, 91
heart-rate 38, 43, 112, 116, 135, 183
Henry Beecher 25
High Density Lipoproteins (HDLs) 90, 91
high-carbohydrate 65, 95, 99, 101, 102, 106
high-fat 99, 109
hippocampus 114, 172
Hippocratic oath 49
hobbies 138, 193
homeostasis 82
homogenisation 75
honesty 144, 206
honourable 206
humility 201
Humphrey, Nicholas 33
hyperglycaemia 97
hypertension 91, 135
hypnosis 48
hypoglycaemia 9, 97, 98, 100

I

iatrogenesis 46
Id 199
Illich, Ivan 46, 48
illness 119, 123, 179, 188
immune system 33, 34, 64, 90, 96, 135

259

income equality 150
indoctrination 11
injury 34, 111, 118, 123, 179, 188
insulin 17, 93, 94, 95, 96, 99, 104, 109, 113
intestine 93
irrationality
    delusional 8, 11
Irritable Bowel Syndrome (IBS) 122
isolation 181

J

Jeffers ,Susan 180
jet lag 134
Jonsson, Gudrun 91
Journal of the American Medical Association (JAMA) 52, 62, 67
judgement 184, 191, 194, 205, 208, 210

K

Katie ,Byron 187
ketogenic diet 104
ketone bodies 104
ketosis 104
Keys, Ancel 64
kidneys 91
kindness 210, 214
Kirsch, Irving 30
Klopfer, Bruno 28
Krauss, Robert 91
Kwaśniewski, Dr. Jan 107

L

labelling 161, 175
Las-Tzu 201
laughter 20, 34, 49, 126, 150, 153, 166, 178
lipase 93, 109

lipogenesis 85
lipolysis 85, 95
liver 88, 90, 95, 104
lobbying 13, 57
Locus Coeruleus 115
loneliness 140
love 163, 214
Low Density Lipoproteins (LDLs) 90, 91, 95
low-calorie 62, 63, 65, 85, 86
low-carbohydrate 62, 63, 64, 66, 86, 95, 96, 98, 99, 104, 106, 107, 109
low-fat 66, 67, 68, 101
low-saturated-fat 68

M

Mannatech 57
margarine 56
marijuana 131, 133
mastitis 74
meat 60, 73, 77, 79, 80, 81, 82, 88, 99
medical care 14
medical industry 40, 48, 148
medical journals 52
medical training 45, 46
meditation 114, 128, 184, 211
melanin 128
melanoma 127
melatonin 133
menopause 136
mental health 81
mesomorphs 105
messages
    continuity 65
    duration 9, 16
    intensity 9, 60, 103
    penetration 9
    repetition 18, 60
    simplicity 9, 17, 69, 90, 106
metabolism 61, 63, 64, 85, 86, 87, 95, 98, 104, 105, 107

milk 17, 55, 56, 61, 70, 74, 75, 77, 81,
    82, 87, 89
mistakes 161, 180, 195
moderation 201, 209
monounsaturated fats 87, 88
morals 203
morphine 23, 25, 42, 114
multiple sclerosis 109, 131

N

National Institute of Health (NIH)
    67
neocortex 156
Nestle, Marion 59
neurogenesis 114
neuroplasticity 130, 142, 158
newspapers 13, 28, 50
nocebo effect 27, 35
nutrigenomics 84
nutrition 45, 48, 54, 59, 60, 70, 81,
    84, 91

O

obesity 61, 62, 65, 85, 86, 94, 96,
    107, 113
Obsessive Compulsive Disorder
    (OCD) 131, 158
oleic acid 88
Olestra 56
omega fatty acids
    omega 3 17, 18, 88
    omega 6 18, 88
optimism 161, 172
organic illness 122
organic 73, 77
osteoarthritis 98
oxytocin 214

P

pain 28, 31, 33, 34, 41, 63, 118, 121, 122,
    182, 192
pancreas 17, 93, 95, 96, 104
panic attacks 116, 183
parasympathetic nervous system 106,
    107, 150
pasteurisation 75
pausing 190
Pennington, Alfred 62
perfectionism 195
pessimism 172
pharmaceutical industry 14, 26, 31, 32,
    35, 39, 46, 50, 52, 67, 89, 133, 148
physicians, See: doctors
pineal gland 133
placebo effect 25, 26, 34
placebo 26, 27, 28, 29, 30, 31, 32, 33, 35,
    131, 172
pleasing others 162
pleasure 144
politicians 5, 16, 67
politics 16
polyunsaturated fats 87, 88
power 7
prefrontal cortex 115
prejudice 193
prevention 39, 40, 45
Price, Weston 80, 81, 97
processed food 55
procrastination 188
Proteases 93
protein 59, 74, 75, 76, 87, 93, 105, 107,
    108
Prozac 30, 32
psychopaths 4, 6, 7, 161, 181
psychopathy 2
psychotherapy 167, 182

R

Reiter, Russell 133

relaxation 126, 128, 132, 144, 161,
   197, 210
religion 138
remorse 3
respect 160
responsibility 164
rest 61, 181, 213
retribution 187

S

Sagan ,Eugene 160
salt 91
saturated fat 64, 66, 67, 87, 88
Schwarzbein, Diana 107
scientific method 19, 21, 22, 24, 62,
   108
Seasonal Affective Disorder (SAD)
   134
self-esteem 119, 146, 160, 161, 163,
   164, 167, 180, 191
self-fulfilling prophecies 28, 35, 36,
   37
self-help 154
sensitivity 180, 195
serotonin 90, 93, 94, 214
Seroxat 32
Sertralin 112
Serzone 32
shoulds and musts 162, 175
side-effects 24, 63, 72, 92
simplicity 11, 16
sleep apnea 117
sleep 34, 41, 42, 132
soil 71, 73, 82
soybeans 18
spiritual 137
sport 111
starches 60
statins 89, 90
status 201
stearic acid 88
Stefansson 80

stomach 17, 59, 91, 92, 93, 101, 122
stress 90, 111, 122, 124, 128, 135, 138,
   182, 187, 214
stretching 118
subconscious 27, 116, 128, 152, 156,
   160, 161, 190, 204, 210
suffering 192
sugar 55, 57, 67, 69, 82, 87, 93, 94, 98,
   101, 102
sun 127
super-ego 199
supermarkets 10, 75, 89
surgery 48
sweeteners 94
sweets 8
sympathetic nervous system 106, 107,
   114
symptoms 15, 20, 21, 24, 39, 41, 42
syndrome X 97
syrup of ipecac 27

T

Tai Chi 111
talking 155, 193, 214
Taoism 144, 201, 204, 209
Taubes, Gary 98
teeth 80, 81, 98
thermodynamics 85
thinking 171
tobacco 93, 132, 135, 149
tonsillectomy 48
traditional methods 148
traditional 20
treatment 39
triglycerides 57, 87, 89, 95
TV 111

U

ultrasound treatment 28
uninhibited 3

UVA 127
UVB 127

V

vagus nerve 92
vegetables 17, 55, 69, 80, 94, 95
Vioxx 52
visual cortex 121
vitamins and minerals 45, 55, 71, 73,
   76, 79, 81, 93
vitamins 93
   vitamin A 42, 76, 88, 93
   vitamin B1 82
   vitamin C 24, 97
   vitamin D 76, 88, 93, 127
   vitamin E 82, 88, 93
   vitamin K 76, 88, 93

W

walking 116, 126, 148
Weeks ,Clare 184
work 137, 148
World Health Organisation (WHO) 88
worry 187
Wrench, G.T. 42

Y

yoga 116

About the author

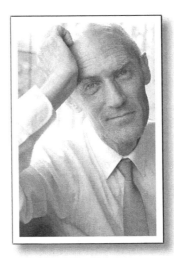

Neil Moffatt was born in the London Borough of Hillingdon in 1957. He moved to Cardiff, South Wales in 1969, his current home. After nearly five enjoyable years as an engineer at BBC Radio in central London, he moved to an 18 year career with IBM and other companies as a systems and application programmer, eventually returning to Wales in 2000.

Health issues saw a move in 2001 to self employment in various guises, most recently as a professional Wedding photographer and author – detailing in this book all that he had learnt about health.

His hobbies have ranged from an obsession with the Chinese game of Go to sport, reading, writing cabinet making, drawing, painting, photography, and design.

neil**moffatt**.co.uk